PANDEMIC PROTECTION

DON COLBERT, MD

SILOAM

Most Charisma House Book Group products are available at special quantity discounts for bulk purchase for sales promotions, premiums, fund-raising, and educational needs. For details, call us at (407) 333-0600 or visit our website at www.charismahouse.com.

PANDEMIC PROTECTION by Don Colbert, MD
Published by Siloam
Charisma Media/Charisma House Book Group
600 Rinehart Road, Lake Mary, Florida 32746

Visit the author's website at divinehealthwellness.com, www.drcolbertbooks.com.

Library of Congress Cataloging-in-Publication Data:
An application to register this book for cataloging has been
submitted to the Library of Congress.
International Standard Book Number: 978-1-62999-901-2
E-book ISBN: 978-1-62999-902-9

This book contains the opinions and ideas of its author. It
is solely for informational and educational purposes and
should not be regarded as a substitute for professional medical
treatment. The nature of your body's health condition is
complex and unique. Therefore, you should consult a health
professional before you begin any new exercise, nutrition, or
supplementation program or if you have questions about your
health. Neither the author nor the publisher shall be liable or
responsible for any loss or damage allegedly arising from any
information or suggestion in this book.

People and names in this book are composites created by the
author from his experiences as a medical doctor. Names and
details of their stories have been changed, and any similarity
between the names and stories of individuals described in this
book and individuals known to readers is purely coincidental.

20 21 22 23 24—987654321
Printed in the United States of America

CONTENTS

INTRODUCTION

THE FLU OUTBREAK was serious—and spreading.

Americans have since grown accustomed to "flu season" bringing an annual variation of the virus. Death rates are typically low and affect mostly the elderly and ailing. But this flu season was proving different.

In New York City, hospitals began to be overwhelmed. Hundreds of thousands were falling ill at the same time. Equipment and beds ran short. In many places, doctors and nurses were nowhere to be found because of the sheer number of people they were tending. A strict quarantine was announced, and yet the death toll continued to rise: ten thousand, twenty thousand, thirty thousand...[1]

While most flus leave behind a trail of temporary discomfort and missed days of work and school, this one was aggressive and merciless. It preyed on young and old alike. In spite of public health measures, it traveled freely through one population and another, respecting no borders, no age, no race.

This time, it seemed, nobody was safe.

In south Philadelphia, streets "stank of rot and excrement." One description put it this way:

> The corpses had backed up at undertakers', filling every area of these establishments and pressing up into living quarters; in hospital morgues overflowing into corridors; in the city morgue overflowing into the street. And they had backed up in homes. They lay on porches, in closets, in corners of the floor, on beds....A wife would lie next to a dead husband, unwilling to move him or leave him. The corpses [were] reminders of death and bringers of terror or grief.[2]

The lungs of people afflicted with the virus filled with fluid, causing blood to hemorrhage from the nose, stomach, and intestines. Their lungs were ripped apart from the inside out as their immune systems attacked the virus—and damaged their own flesh in the process.[3]

Every worker in New York City wore a mask. In some cities life seemed to have stopped altogether. Public meetings were banned; churches, schools, and theaters all closed.[4]

As familiar as these scenes may sound, this is not a description of any recent pandemic, nor a film script or imaginary scenario. This is a true account of what happened in 1918–20 when the Spanish flu swept the globe. Before it was done, it claimed tens of millions of lives and was the worst natural calamity of the twentieth century.

PRESENT-DAY PROTECTION

Pandemics have been with humanity for thousands of years. Viruses and other germs wield massive influence over life on earth. Governments and kings may rule, but there are times when pandemics overrule them all.

As serious as recent pandemics have been, humans recently have been spared the worst that history has to offer. Some of this is due to improved overall health in Western populations, and to quick action by public authorities to isolate new virulent infections. But the pandemic gun is already being reloaded, and it's only a matter of time before the next potential outbreak finds a foothold somewhere—an Asian market; an African village; an American community—and joins the pantheon of pandemics in history that shape lives, change societies, and even topple empires.

The good news is that we don't need to be at the mercy of pandemics. As individuals, cities, and nations we have the power to rewrite our future when a virus or other invader comes knocking. The answer is not just in vaccines, which can be helpful, but in the personal preparation we perform right now to build our defenses through a lifestyle of health and wellness. Medical science has shown over and over again that victory goes to the prepared—to those whose bodies, minds, and spirits are firmly grounded in health-giving practices and habits.

This will certainly require some changes on your part—but they will be worth it.

You can help prevent the next pandemic from harming you, your family, your community and nation. This book will show you how.

CHAPTER 1

LESSONS FROM PANDEMICS PAST

INFLUENZA HAS LIKELY been around for more than two thousand years. The word *influenza* originated in sixteenth-century Italy and was later applied to epidemics, with the idea being that pandemics were attributed to the influence of the stars.[1]

People later shortened it to "flue" and "flu"—and so the medieval term remains the official one for what we now know is caused not by stars or planets but by microscopic invaders.[2]

All influenza viruses come from birds. Their extraordinarily rapid mutation rate at some point allowed them to jump from birds to mammals. The virus can adapt to birds, swine, and humans, forming a new variant that can spread rapidly. A virus is nothing more than a (usually) spherical membrane that contains the eight genes that define what the virus is.[3]

Lacking sufficient genes to reproduce itself, a virus enters a cell where it hides from our immune system and hijacks the cell, causing it to produce many viruses. These then burst the cell and infect other cells. These newly created viruses repeat the process until our bodies stop them or until we die.[4]

Compared to viruses, bacteria are rather unsophisticated and usually easier for our bodies to identify and deal with. They can still do real damage, but scientists still have not found a way to combat viruses that is as effective as something like penicillin.[5]

Estimates tell us every year there are one billion influenza infections worldwide, with 290,000 to 650,000 deaths. Of these, the United States experiences up to 45 million cases and tens of thousands of deaths every year.[6]

The seasonal flu has a fatality rate of less than 1 percent, and experts say the rate is closer to 0.1 percent.[7]

But while we know much more than we ever have about this tiny menace, we still don't know how to defeat it completely. According to a paper published by the National Institutes of Health, "Major influenza epidemics show no predictable periodicity or pattern, and all differ from one another."[8]

That makes them a constantly moving target. The virus' ability to mutate rapidly, along with the global extent of human travel in the modern world, exposes us to more dangerous infections from around the world than ever before. Author Joel Fuhrman puts it this way:

> We are routinely in airports and jets crowded with world travelers who have come in contact with exotic and newly created microbes, and we are in schools and hospitals with bacteria circulating that have developed antibiotic resistance. Scientists suggest that environmental, social, and nutritional changes have helped trigger an unprecedented explosion of infection: more than thirty-five new infectious diseases have burst upon the world in the past thirty years. The U.S. death rate from infectious diseases is now double what it was in 1980, up to 170,000 annually.... Once a disease takes hold these days, it tends to be globalized quickly by travel and trade.[9]

For example, it took just six weeks for SARS (severe acute respiratory syndrome) to spread worldwide in November 2002, carried by unsuspecting travelers. "It set a record for speed of continent-to-continent transmission," Fuhrman writes.[10]

So while science has caught up with facts about what causes influenza and other plagues, permanent solutions still lag behind.

Let's briefly trace the ugly history of some of the worst pandemics the human race has ever experienced.

THE BLACK DEATH

For three hundred years, from 1348 to 1665, a recurring plague rose up every twenty years and decimated the city of London. Some estimate that with each new wave of epidemic, 20 percent of the men, women, and children living in London were killed. There were forty such plagues over three centuries causing almost incomprehensible, repeat destruction and grief.[11]

The practice of quarantining began during the fourteenth century when port authorities in the Venetian-controlled port of Ragusa required ships arriving from infected ports to sit at anchor for forty days before landing to prove that the sailors weren't sick. Nobody knew what caused the Black Death, but they knew it had something to do with proximity.[12] The term *quarantine* was born from the Italian *quaranta giorni*, which means "forty days."[13]

The first laws to separate and isolate the sick were instituted in the early 1500s, when plague-stricken homes in England were identified by a bale of hay attached to a pole outside. People who had infected family members were made to carry a white pole when they went into public.[14]

The Great Plague of 1665 culminated London's afflictions, killing one hundred thousand of that city's residents in just seven months. It began in the late spring, and by the fall, roughly seven thousand people were dying every week. Residents had to navigate around corpses lying in the streets, and people read the grim weekly death tolls posted in public places. King Charles II halted all public gatherings, including funerals, in 1666.[15]

One article puts it this way:

Already, theaters had been shut down in London, and licensing curtailed for new pubs. Oxford and Cambridge closed.... Public servants called searchers ferreted out new cases of plague, and quarantined sick people along with everyone who shared their homes. People called warders painted a red cross on the doors of quarantined homes, alongside a paper notice that read "LORD HAVE MERCY UPON US."...

The government supplied food to the housebound. After 40 days, warders painted over the red crosses with white crosses, ordering residents to sterilize their homes with lime. Doctors believed that the bubonic plague was caused by "smells" in the air, so cleaning was always recommended. They had no idea that it was also a good way to get rid of the ticks and fleas that actually spread the contagion....

But there was some good advice, too. During the Great Plague, shopkeepers asked customers to drop their coins in dishes of vinegar to sterilize them, using the 1600s version of hand sanitizer.[16]

The isolation and other measures worked, and England never experienced such a plague again. At least, not in that form.

SMALLPOX

From the sixth century onward, and perhaps even earlier, smallpox was a dreaded killer in Europe, where it stole the lives of three of every ten people it infected and left the rest with pockmark scars.[17] The viral infection was accompanied by a fever and distinctive skin rash that began on the tongue and in the mouth and then spread quickly to the face, arms, legs, and the rest of the body. By the fourth day of infection the sores became pustules, which then began to crust and scab over. Three weeks after the rash first appeared, the scabs would fall off, and the damage would have been done—if the person remained alive.[18]

As great as the toll was in Europe, it became almost unimaginable in the New World across the Atlantic. Smallpox arrived in the Americas in the fifteenth century with European sailors and did its worst damage, killing up to 95 percent of the indigenous population in the United States and Mexico in one century.[19]

Nearly two centuries after a vaccine was first discovered, in 1980 the World Health Organization announced that smallpox had become the first virus to be completely eradicated from the face of the earth by vaccine.

That last natural outbreak of smallpox occurred in the US in 1949.[20]

Those of us alive today have never dreaded smallpox as our ancestors did. By God's grace it has been resigned to history books.

CHOLERA

In the nineteenth century, cholera, a bacterial intestinal illness resulting from feces-contaminated drinking water, killed tens of thousands in England. The bacteria worked quickly, bringing death to some within hours of first symptoms. Scientists at the time believed cholera was spread by foul air known as a *miasma*. But a British doctor named John Snow believed differently. In 1854 a London mother washed her baby's diaper and dumped the water in a cesspit near a town well on Broad Street, creating a mini-epidemic that killed 616 people.

> "Within 250 yards of the spot where Cambridge Street joins Broad Street there were upwards of 500 fatal attacks of cholera in 10 days," Dr. Snow wrote. "As soon as I

5

became acquainted with the situation and extent of this irruption (sic) of cholera, I suspected some contamination of the water of the much-frequented street-pump in Broad Street."[21]

Snow investigated hospital records and morgue reports to track the precise locations of deadly outbreaks. He created a geographic chart of cholera deaths over a ten-day period and found a cluster of five hundred fatal infections surrounding the Broad Street pump, a popular city well for drinking water.[22]

"According to Snow's records, the keeper of one coffee shop in the neighborhood who served glasses of water from the Broad Street pump along with meals said she knew of nine of her customers who had contracted cholera." Just as important, Snow discovered a nearby workhouse that had no cases of cholera among its more than five hundred inmates because the prison had its own well.[23]

Snow convinced skeptical local officials to remove the pump handle on the Broad Street drinking well, rendering it unusable. Infections dried up immediately.[24]

Cholera is no longer prevalent in developed countries, but it remains a dangerous problem in countries lacking proper sewage treatment and access to clean drinking water.

THE SPANISH FLU

Then there was the Spanish flu, which almost certainly took more than fifty million lives, and perhaps one hundred million lives, worldwide. The flu was not Spanish at all but received that title because it was widely reported in Spanish newspapers, which were not facing wartime censorship. Like the recent COVID-19 outbreak, but to a much greater degree, the Spanish flu killed people in their prime—their twenties and thirties—not just the elderly. "Roughly half of those who died were young men and women in the prime of their life, in their twenties and thirties....As many as 8 to 10 percent of all young adults then living may have been killed by the virus....Influenza killed more people in a year than the Black Death of the Middle Ages killed in a century,"—most of them in the last few months of 1918.[25]

In Philadelphia, the number of bodies exceeded the number of available graves, and victims were buried without coffins in mass graves.[26]

The virus accelerated death for those suffering from cancer, heart disease, stroke, tuberculosis, and other chronic ailments, and its grim work depressed the average life expectancy in the United States by more than ten years.[27]

In today's numbers the Spanish flu would have taken 1.75 million American lives. Many of those lost were serving in World War I in close quarters with other troops where "the stresses of combat and war, and their malnourished state all contributed to their depressed immune system function, increasing their susceptibility."[28]

The 1918 virus was so lethal at its beginning that over time its mutations actually made it less lethal.[29]

Its brief but potent reign of terror ended in 1920.

ASIAN OUTBREAKS

A major outbreak in the 1950s killed between one million and two million people. In 1957 the first wave of the Asian flu hit children, while the second wave mostly affected the elderly. "The Centers for Disease Control and Prevention notes that the disease spread rapidly and was reported in Singapore in February 1957, Hong Kong in April 1957, and the coastal cities of the United States in the summer of 1957."[30] "The medical community was able to identify that pandemic more quickly because of improvements in scientific technology, according to the US Centers for Disease Control."[31]

Ten years later, in early 1968, "a flu pandemic surfaced in Hong Kong," killing around 33,800 people in six months, "making it one of the mildest pandemics of the 20th century."[32]

In 1997 a potential outbreak was averted: a Hong Kong virus that killed six of eighteen people it infected was prevented from adapting to people by public health authorities who had every chicken in Hong Kong—more than a million of them—slaughtered. Wholesale slaughter was the solution again in 2003 in Europe when a new virus appeared in poultry farms in the Netherlands, Belgium, and Germany. "This virus infected eighty-two people and killed one, and it also infected pigs," writes Barry. "Public health authorities killed nearly thirty million poultry and some swine."[33]

SWINE FLU (H1N1 FLU, 2009)

The first influenza pandemic of the twenty-first century, the 2009 swine (H1N1) flu, was caused by a new strain of virus that originated in Mexico. "In one year, the virus infected as many as 1.4 billion people across the globe and killed between 151,700 and 575,400 people, according to the CDC."[34] "It was the first pandemic for which many Member States had developed comprehensive pandemic plans describing the public health measures to be taken, aimed at reducing illness and fatalities. For the first time, pandemic vaccine was developed, produced and deployed in multiple countries during the first year of the pandemic."[35]

> The World Health Organization...called the swine flu outbreak spreading around the world a "public health emergency of international concern."[36]

Swine flu "primarily affected children and young adults, and 80% of the deaths were in people younger than 65, the CDC reported. That was unusual, considering that most strains of flu viruses, including those that cause seasonal flu, cause the highest percentage of deaths in people ages 65 and older. But in the case of the swine flu, older people seemed to have already built up enough immunity to the group of viruses" that swine flu belonged to.[37]

SARS, EBOLA, ZIKA

SARS—a cousin to COVID-19, and itself a coronavirus—was very virulent, but was successfully contained. It's amazing that health community leaders kept SARS from going pandemic. According to the World Health Organization, 8,400 people were infected with SARS, and about 900 eventually died during the outbreak.[38]

From 2014 to 2016, Ebola ravaged West Africa, causing 11,325 deaths.[39] Ebola is a viral hemorrhagic fever spread through direct contact with bodily fluids such as blood or other fluids from infected individuals. It is caused by the Ebola virus. The Zika virus epidemic in South America and Central America was spread through mosquitoes, and could be sexually transmitted. It could also be transmitted by a pregnant mother to her fetus. After a few cases showed up in the US in 2016 and 2017, the virus disappeared from our shores.[40]

The flu doesn't need a fancy name or nonstop news cycles to continue its deadly work. In 2017 to 2018, the worst flu season on record in the US outside of a pandemic, more than sixty thousand Americans died.[41] And yet virtually no one paid attention, beyond those affected.

COVID-19

The official name of the virus is SARS-CoV-2, which stands for severe acute respiratory syndrome coronavirus 2. Most people who lived through it call it simply "coronavirus."

COVID-19 caught much of the world off guard. Within weeks normal life became strange and surreal. Times Square in New York City was empty. Hospitals and morgues in some cities were full. Bodies were put in freezers temporarily.

The virus didn't act like "normal" influenzas. It seemed to afflict young adults and the old. "We're seeing younger patients, one a 29-year-old, some in their 40s, 50s," Dr. Adam Jarrett, chief medical officer of Holy Name Medical Center in Teaneck New Jersey, told NBC News, also stating patients' ages were younger than expected.[42]

The virus seemed hardier than others. One fifty-two-year-old woman's infection "was linked to her sitting in a seat at a church that had been occupied earlier in the day by two tourists who showed no symptoms but later fell ill, investigators said after they reviewed closed-circuit camera recordings of church services."[43]

And "a startlingly high number of people infected with the new coronavirus may not show symptoms, the director of the Centers for Disease Control and Prevention said, complicating efforts to predict the pandemic's course and strategies to mitigate its spread.... For example," the *New York Times* reported, "as many as 18 percent of people infected with the virus on the Diamond Princess cruise ship never developed symptoms, according to one analysis. A team in Hong Kong suggests that from 20 to 40 percent of transmissions in China occurred before symptoms appeared. The high level of covert spread may help explain why the novel coronavirus is the first virus that is not an influenza virus to set off a pandemic."[44] COVID-19 is much more contagious than the flu.

- A small study showed that people with type A blood were more likely to get it, while people with type O were less so.[45]
- Men were more susceptible to it than women.[46]
- And if you got it once, you could get it again, as a few people recovered from COVID-19 and were then reinfected.[47]

According to the World Health Organization, "With each pandemic, researchers, public health experts and international organizations have gained a better understanding of the complexity and dynamics of influenza pandemics. With the improvement of surveillance and reporting systems, more data and characteristics of viruses can be documented than was possible a decade ago."[48]

But there is something more we can do than cheer for the scientists, doctors, and public health personnel to save us from pandemics. We are not doomed to fall victim to each passing plague. No! God has given us the tools and the wisdom to determine our own destiny. Dr. Joel Fuhrman puts it this way:

> What if science advanced to the point where it became possible to become almost totally resistant to colds, influenza, and other infections—and if you did "catch" something, you bounced back to wellness within twenty-four hours? What if we could prevent the complications of viral and bacterial exposures and keep them as minor annoyances that never evolved into more dangerous infections? What if it were possible to develop Super Immunity to infections?...What if we found out how to build

immune defenses with proper nutrition to develop Super Immunity?[49]

I agree with Fuhrman and go beyond his advice. I believe there is a way to achieve a high level of preparation for any pandemic by building up our immune systems in advance. This involves having the right diet, sleep regimen, exercise habits, supplements, a peaceful mindset, common sense measures, and a firm reliance on God's Word and its many promises of health and protection.

I have seen it work in the lives of others, and in my own life. Practical pandemic protection is for you as well.

CHAPTER 2

IMMUNE SYSTEM 101

A SILENT WAR AGAINST pandemics is taking place around the clock, every day of our lives. This war occurs not in government labs or hospitals. Rather, it is happening inside of you and me, even at this very moment. Within every human body on the planet God has installed the best defense system against viruses, bacteria, and plagues of all kinds. This defensive team is called the immune system, and it is brilliantly effective and capable of adapting to meet new threats.

Without our immune systems, pandemics would have finished off the human race centuries ago. Our magnificent, built-in response mechanisms speak not only to God's incredible wisdom and infinite ability but to His care and concern for each human being. Let's look for a moment at the amazing system God put inside of us to protect us from harmful invaders.

LAYERS OF PROTECTION

Every day our bodies are under siege from viruses, bacteria, fungi, and other opportunistic "germs" that want to prey upon us for their own advantage. Like our country's armed services, our immune system has several branches that specialize in defending our bodies in different ways. One branch is a generalized force that fights against any foreign invader. Others are like cellular SEALs that specialize in targeted warfare against specific opponents. Some immune system cells are ground troops doing hand-to-hand combat, some function like snipers at a distance, some are reconnaissance experts, and some work the supply lines.

Warding off disease from our bodies begins at the simple,

mechanical level—the physical barriers of skin and mucous membranes. By far, most would-be invaders stop here. They simply cannot get through the "walls" of our skin and mucous membranes. Every day this physical system repels countless attempted attacks without our even knowing it.

THE WAR INSIDE

When the physical barrier is breached, we find that we develop a swollen infection at the site of a cut, or a persistent cough, or something worse like a viral or bacterial infection in our bloodstream. When viruses and bacteria pass through the skin or mucous barriers, it becomes an inside game, and here is where the genius of our immune systems really shines.

Everyone possesses two broad types of immune system: *innate* and *acquired* (or *adaptive*). Every person is born with an innate immune response. Each of us then uniquely develops an acquired immune response based on the invaders to which we are exposed.

The innate immune response is general and highly sensitive, recognizing that something that is not part of our bodies is present, and alerting the rest of the system to pay attention and get to work. Your body can recognize millions of different invaders. The acquired system then kicks in to specifically identify and react to that invader. Your immune system remembers and recognizes every bacterium and virus it has encountered before, and can effectively repel it should it attack again.[1]

These branches of our immune systems work together like little armies—almost literally. Some cells are trained to attack any foreign invaders. Some attack only specific types of foreign invaders. Some "paint targets" like elite armed forces do when pointing lasers at enemy buildings or encampments for a missile strike. These cells smear antigens with a protein that other "killer" cells recognize as a message to destroy that cell. Other cells open passageways for these killer cells to pass through. Still others send alerts to other branches of the immune system to tell them where to go and what to do.

Author John Barry calls the immune system "an extraordinarily complex, intricate, and interwoven combination of various kinds of white blood cells, antibodies, enzymes, toxins, and other proteins. The key to the immune system is its ability to distinguish what belongs in the body, 'self,' from what does not belong, 'nonself.'"[2]

He continues:

> The recognition of a foreign antigen also sets off a parallel chain of events as the body releases enzymes. Some of these affect the entire body, for example, raising its temperature and causing fever. Others directly attack and kill the target. Still others serve as chemical messengers, summoning white blood cells to areas of invasion or dilating capillaries so killer cells can exit the bloodstream at the point of attack. Swelling, redness, and fever are all side effects of the release of these chemicals. All this together is called the "immune response," and once the immune system is mobilized it is formidable indeed. But all this takes time. The delay can allow infections to gain a foothold in the body.[3]

Let's look a little closer at your body's immune response to the presence of an invader.

FIRST RESPONDERS AND SPECIALISTS

A type of white blood cell called a *granulocyte* is your body's first responder. Granulocyte cells don't have memory of what has invaded before, and their methods of attack are not very refined:

when you scrape yourself, or some invading entity or debris is introduced beneath your skin, the granulocytes gather there en masse and begin to "eat" every non-self item in sight. They do this by digesting foreign particles with poisons the granulocyte itself produces, including hydrogen peroxide, nitric oxide, and hypochlorite, which is the active ingredient in bleach. Granulocytes hold the fort until more-sophisticated and trained responders arrive. The granulocytes usually die throwing themselves into battle.[4]

Another type of white blood cell then arrives, the macrophage. Macrophages circulate in the blood and enter the tissues when there is an infection. There are far fewer macrophages in our blood than there are granulocytes, but the macrophage is more of a specialist. It bumps into an invader such as a bacterium or virus, touches it with antenna-like proteins that radiate from its membrane, and identifies specific characteristics of the invader. It then attacks with the same chemicals the granulocytes produced, but tailored to the invader's characteristics. The chemicals a macrophage produces are known collectively as *cytokines*, and these can cause fever and sleepiness in our bodies. Cytokines also play an important role in limiting the immune response to the appropriate level for the threat.[5]

While they seem to perform the same function, macrophages are better communicators than are granulocytes. Macrophages spread the word to other parts of the immune system, especially T cells, which are even more specific and powerful. Amazingly the macrophages take little parts of the now-dead invaders and place them on cuplike structures on the macrophages' outer membranes. They then share this information with a certain type of T cell. Only a very few T cells recognize what the invader is by that information, but when they do, they launch a specific attack against it by reproducing many cells that recognize the particular antigen, and dispersing them throughout your body by way of the bloodstream.[6]

THYMUS

How did T cells get so smart? They went to school, quite literally, in an organ called the thymus. The thymus is perhaps the most important organ involved in your immune reaction. It is located in front of the heart and is the military academy where T cells, which are born in our bone marrow and move to the thymus, learn what to fight. In the thymus each T cell is shown different antigens (an antigen is any "non-self" entity in our bodies, usually harmful). If the T cell recognizes the antigen it is presented with, and reacts to it as to an invader, the T cell moves on to further training. If it fails to respond to a foreign antigen, it is destroyed, because it is useless in an immune response.

The T cell is then presented with parts of the organism itself—your own body. If the T cell treats this like an antigen, the T cell is destroyed—and good thing. Otherwise it would attack your own body as if your body were the invader. This is the kind of reaction that causes autoimmune diseases.

When a T cell passes all its tests, it is sent to the front lines—the bloodstream—to look for invaders. The thymus, then, is the site of our immune system's most critical preparations.

During an attack, another type of cell, called the B cell, performs a different function. B cells create antibodies tailored to the specific antigen, then go about their job in several different ways. One thing B cells do is coat the invader with an antigen that attracts macrophages and granulocytes, which then destroy the "bad guy." B cells also cover antigens with a kind of glue that causes them to stick together, making them an easy target for other immune responders to attack and kill. Yet a third strategy is to coat a bacterium or virus with an antibody that prevents it from attaching to other cells.[7]

Your B cells also "remember" the invader and record its characteristics in their genes.[8]

We are still learning about the brilliant intricacies of the immune system, but what we know already about its scope and complexity is simply breathtaking.

BACKUP SYSTEMS IN PLACE

Redundancy is built into the immune system so that if one system or immunity-related organ is lost or damaged, the other systems and organs can pick up its functions.

During a pandemic larger numbers of people are attacked and infected by the same virus or bacteria for which much of the human population has not developed antibodies. This occurred with devastating effect, as I mentioned earlier, when Europeans began colonizing the Americas. The Incas, Aztecs, and other Native American peoples had no previous exposure to smallpox and virtually no ability to defend themselves from it. Mexico went from a population of eleven million to about one million.[9]

When a virus mutates enough, the human immune system cannot recognize it. If a virus is novel enough that nobody's immune system has encountered it before, it can spread through a population like wildfire. That is the definition of a pandemic.

Unfortunately, as we age, the thymus atrophies (shrivels up), which is why people over the age of sixty are more susceptible to illness. They can't help it; their immune systems are on the black diamond slope downhill—that is, until we begin to strengthen them with the knowledge, supplements, and lifestyle habits that empower the thymus and other important immunity-related entities in our bodies.

Our God-given immune systems are beautiful and powerful. The cells that fight foreign invaders are the true heroes in any pandemic. But like everything, this system requires our support to function at the peak level God intended. When we choose to walk in a basic lifestyle of health, we give our "troops" everything they need to fight against pandemic diseases and run-of-the-mill infections.

When our immune systems are strong, we enjoy a high level of protection—no matter what contagion is sweeping the globe.

CHAPTER 3

THE BEST DIET TO BOOST THE IMMUNE SYSTEM

As our inner defense forces quietly fight our most important physical battles, we must do our part to create supply lines that help them win the conflicts. A major aspect of those supply lines is our diet and the health of our gut.

Many people seem to have good supply lines because they eat plenty of food, but in reality they are sending junk to their front lines. Our bodies need specific supplies called nutrients. What good would it do to send ice cream and cupcakes to men in the heat of battle? Or to airdrop notebooks and pens to them? They would respond, "We don't need this stuff; we need more bullets and grenades!"

In a similar way, many of us give our bodies junk food they don't need, which depletes us of nutrients, and which takes energy to process and dispose of. Meanwhile our bodies are sending messages back to the supply source saying, "Send us nutrients! We have battles to fight, and we're running out of support."

IMMUNITY TAKES GUTS

A good diet supports immune function in another way as well that many people are unaware of: by giving us good gut health. Gut health is the foundation of all health. The ancient physician Hippocrates (c. 460–c. 370 BC) is often attributed with saying, "All disease begins in the gut." Many of today's medical experts are coming to the same conclusion—based on scientific research.

Few people realize that approximately 75 percent of your body's total immune cells are found in your gut! Your body holds about

100 trillion bacteria, and one drop of fluid from your colon contains more than a billion of these bacteria.[1]

These account for 90 percent of the total number of cells in your body![2] Yes, that means only 10 percent of your cells are human.

Author Robynne Chutkan writes that "microbial health is one of the factors that determines who survives potentially deadly viruses."[3]

According to scientists at the National Institutes of Health, "these complex communities of microbes that include bacteria, fungi, viruses and other microbial and eukaryotic species provide a tremendous enzymatic capability and play a fundamental role in controlling many aspects of host physiology. Over the past few years, the field of immunology has been revolutionized by the growing understanding of the fundamental role of the microbiota in the induction, education, and function of the mammalian immune system."[4]

In other words, our guts not only digest and eliminate food—they literally help to train our immune systems![5]

Our guts actually instruct our immune systems which bacteria are bad, and help immune cells to grow![6]

Noted neurologist Dr. David Perlmutter went so far as to say, "90 percent of all known human illness can be traced back to an unhealthy gut. And we can say for sure that just as disease begins in the gut, so too does health and vitality."[7]

Dr. Fuhrman says that "research has shown that the influenza virus also exhibits increased virulence in a nutritionally deficient host, allowing multiple changes in the viral genome. In other words, your everyday flu can mutate and become able to cause more serious damage to the lungs and other parts of the body."[8]

According to an article published by scientists at the NIH, "The immune system is not only controlled by its symbiotic relationship with the microbiota but is also exquisitely sensitive to the nutritional status of the host. Evidence now exists for a multi-directional interaction between the diet, immune system and commensal microflora."[9]

I agree with the way Dr. Fuhrman puts it:

> The nutritional status of the host is critical in permitting or preventing viral and bacterial infections.... Nutritional inadequacies in the host allow the modification of viruses into more virulent or dangerous forms.... When the body is deprived of nutrients, viral infections can cause serious, even fatal diseases that don't occur when deficiency is not present. Immunity, when optimized, can ward off infection; and if infection does occur, it is much more likely to have a harmless outcome.... The most effective artillery we have to protect ourselves against the potentially damaging effects of influenza and other infectious diseases is nutritional excellence.[10]

Unfortunately "nutritional excellence" does not exactly describe the normal American's diet, which does more to weaken resistance to infections than to strengthen it. Less than 5 percent of the average American's total calories come from fresh fruits, vegetables, seeds, and nuts. About half of our vegetable consumption in America is white potato products, which includes fries and chips![11]

If you maintain your gut in a healthy condition, your body and immune system will thrive more. Let's look at simple dietary ways to powerfully restore and maintain immunity-supporting gut health.

THE GUT ZONE DIET—SIMPLIFIED

Let's make our goals simple. What I call the Gut Zone Diet requires that we do two things:

1. Feed the good: The basis of this diet is raw and cooked vegetables, supported by other yummy foods that may surprise you. It also includes things the good bacteria in your gut want, such as probiotics, prebiotics, polyphenols, fiber, and resistant starches. We'll get to these later.

2. Starve the bad: The Gut Zone diet avoids, minimizes, or eliminates sugars, starches, carbs, dairy, artificial sweeteners, and saturated fats. Let's go ahead and start with the bad news—stuff your gut hates.

Enemy #1: Gluten

The most common, and probably most dangerous, enemy to your gut is gluten. Gluten is the protein found in wheat, barley, and rye, as well as most breads, pastas, bagels, pretzels, cereals, cakes, cookies, and in most processed foods. It is possible that virtually everyone may have a negative, albeit undetected reaction to gluten, which can cause lasting damage without you even knowing it.[12]

That means your gut may not be as healthy as you think, and gluten may be one culprit. Two specific gluten proteins cause the most inflammation and damage: glutenins and gliadins. Without going into the why and how, I counsel my patients to wean themselves off gluten as a way of healing the gut and boosting its effectiveness in supporting our immune responses.[13]

Enemy #2: High-Sugar, High-Carb Diet

The second greatest cause of inflammation is a high-sugar, high-carb diet. Think about it: in a sugary environment, bacteria usually grow unchecked. It is no different when we put that sugar in our intestines! The "bad" bacteria feast and multiply. It's no wonder that eating too much sugar and carbs gives us stomachaches. Our gut is literally crying out, "Stop! You're harming your own health!"

Most people don't know that carbohydrates spike blood sugar levels, and high blood sugar levels help throw the body's bacteria levels out of balance and fuel inflammation. It is this imbalance that leads to increased food sensitivities. I believe this is why sugar has been shown to weaken the immune system. When you eat 100 grams of sugar, your white blood cells are 40 percent less effective at killing microbes for up to five hours.[14]

Is that ice cream sandwich really worth compromising your immune response? I don't think so!

Enemy #3: Dairy

Cow's milk stands as one of the top food allergies around the world. People who are lactose intolerant are not adequately digesting the milk sugar called lactose. Lactose in these people usually causes abdominal bloating and diarrhea, which distresses the gut in many people. Dairy also usually inflames the GI tract of many of my patients.

Unfortunately our bodies are dumb—they usually crave the very foods that inflame them! Dairy—and specifically the protein called casein—usually inflames the gut, congests the sinuses and nasal passages, creates mucus, may cause snoring, and may fuel arthritis, among other things.

I recommend that people minimize their dairy intake to see if it makes them feel better. Or try milks that have A2 beta-casein, which may be easier to digest.[15]

It is possible you have learned to live with a level of inflammation in the gut that is caused by dairy. If so, your body is not running at optimal levels—and that includes your immune system.

Enemy #4: Saturated Fats

It is well known that saturated fats don't do us much good at all and are linked with all kinds of health problems, including heart disease. Now we know that saturated fats from things like butter, cheese, coconut oil, cream, and fatty meats inflame the gut by increasing levels of LPS (lipopolysaccharide). You can read more about this in my book *The Gut Zone*. In short, LPS can stimulate the innate immune system to react with a local or systemic inflammatory response, causing increased intestinal permeability or causing inflammation in joints (arthritis), in the brain (causing depression, fatigue, forgetfulness), and throughout our bodies. LPS has been found to raise the levels of a protein found at higher levels in Alzheimer's and Parkinson's sufferers.[16]

Saturated fat causes us to absorb a lot of LPS, and the inflammatory response can be disastrous long-term for our immune system and health. Keep your total saturated fat intake to 10 percent or less to avoid this source of inflammation. It's interesting to note that medium-chain triglycerides from coconuts do not raise LPS levels but coconut oil does.

THE GOOD

Good gut health is not too complicated or too difficult to achieve. And because the entire body is connected to the gut, it is imperative that we get our gut healthy as the basis of every other lifestyle habit we want to implement. Feeling good at the gut level is the beginning from which everything else will follow.[17]

Cruci-fy Your Diet

My top recommendation for almost everybody is to eat more cruciferous vegetables, which are the most powerful anti-cancer foods in existence, and the most micronutrient dense of all vegetables.[18] Examples of cruciferous vegetables are kale, cabbage, brussels sprouts, collards, broccoli, cauliflower, and turnips. The flower petals of these veggies are in the shape of a cross, and so they are aptly named "cross-bearer" in Latin.

Dr. Fuhrman writes that "all vegetables contain protective micronutrients and phytochemicals, but cruciferous vegetables have a unique chemical composition: they have sulfur-containing compounds that are responsible for their pungent or bitter flavors. When their cell walls are broken by blending or chopping, a chemical reaction occurs that converts these sulfur-containing compounds into isothiocyanates (ITCs)—an array of compounds with proven and powerful immune-boosting effects and anticancer activity. . . . Recent studies have shown that these ITCs are important in enabling interferon responsiveness which serves as a potent immune system stimulator to attack microbes such as viruses. Specifically, these ITCs have been shown to increase the immune system's cell-killing capacity and heightened resistance to viral infection, with impressive results."[19]

I try to eat a cruciferous veggie every day. The good news is that cauliflower chips count! I snack all the time on macadamia nuts and cauliflower chips. My wife thinks I'm crazy, but I love them. I buy them in packs of six.

Try cruciferous vegetables in creative ways. Steam them, sauté them, boil them, put them in soups, or eat them raw. I experiment with them in all different ways. I use broccoli, kale, cauliflower, and other cruciferous vegetables in my "immune-boosting soups," along with curry; low-fat, low-sugar coconut milk; garlic; onions; and chicken or organic, lean grass-fed beef once or twice a week. Once it's stopped boiling for a bit, I add two tablespoons of avocado or olive oil, which gives me healthy fats, which are good for the immune system and lower cholesterol.

I also like to steam cruciferous vegetables, because they're gas-producing and can be hard to digest. I find that steaming them makes them not as mushy, and it helps me to chew and digest them better. See if it works for you—but whatever you do, start majoring on these amazingly healthy vegetables.

Go Nuts

I also eat lots of nuts and some seeds, such as almonds, chestnuts, flaxseeds, hazelnuts, macadamia nuts, pecans, pine nuts, pistachios, psyllium seeds or husks, and walnuts. Peanuts and cashews are not nuts; peanuts are legumes, and cashews are seeds. Small amounts of coconut are fine, but I encourage you to avoid too much coconut oil or cream, since it is very high in saturated fat. I like what Dr. Fuhrman shares about nuts, my favorite foods:

> There has never been a study that showed any negative health outcomes from consuming these natural, high-fat, whole plant foods. In fact, the studies all show positive health benefits and conclude that these foods should be an important part of a well-rounded diet.[20]

Good Carbs

Sweet potatoes, yams, yucca, taro root, cassava, jicama, green mangos, green bananas, and millet bread are gut-healing carbs. Other good choices are berries, pressure-cooked beans and peas, and occasional steel-cut oatmeal. Even small amounts of basmati rice—a portion about the size of a tennis ball—are fine. I also enjoy lime cassava chips as a snack, which can be ordered online.

See? I told you it's not complicated.

GET GOOD BACTERIA GOING

Now that you know there are trillions of good bacteria in your gut, and that the gut helps to regulate our immune responses, you will want to make specific effort to feed those champions! One very important way to do this is with probiotic foods. *Probiotic* means it contains good bacteria that improve the health of your gut. Probiotics can be beneficial when viruses spread and cause pandemics. A recent double-blind, randomized controlled scientific study found that "the consumption of probiotics significantly reduced the incidence of upper respiratory infection...and flu-like symptoms."[21]

You can take probiotics as supplements in liquid, pill, or powder form, but probiotics are also found in many different foods and side dishes, such as the following:

- Yogurt—with active or live cultures (goat milk or coconut yogurt preferred)
- Kefir—a fermented milk (goat milk or coconut kefir preferred)
- Sauerkraut—a fermented cabbage
- Tempeh—a fermented soybean patty
- Kimchi—a spicy, fermented Korean dish
- Miso—a fermented Japanese soybean paste

- Kombucha—a tea fermented with sugar, lactic acid bacteria, and yeast
- Pickles—fermented and salty cucumbers
- Traditional buttermilk—fermented dairy drink (prefer goat milk buttermilk)
- Natto—fermented Japanese soybean product
- Select cheeses—Gouda, mozzarella, cheddar, cottage (prefer feta cheese)[22]

Author Giulia Enders writes that "probiotics have a relatively short shelf life in your gut. They are highly effective, but over time they will mostly disappear. That is why continued use of probiotics is necessary and effective."[23]

I usually put my patients on at least one to two probiotic capsules a day and sometimes more. Sometimes I will use two to four different types of probiotics, depending on the severity of their gut problems. I will say more about this in the chapter on supplements.

Author Raphael Kellman wisely instructs that as you work to daily include probiotics in your diet, keep in mind that it is good to shake things up a bit. Rotating probiotics after six months is recommended to keep your gut's "microbiome diverse and healthy."[24]

FEEDING THE COLONIES

Other gut- and immunity-enhancing foods are prebiotics. While probiotics are living organisms, prebiotics are the foods those organisms eat, usually fiber. Fiber comes in two different forms: soluble and insoluble. Your body needs both. Soluble fiber dissolves in your GI tract, absorbs water, and helps with digestion. Insoluble fiber is undigestible by humans, meaning that unlike proteins, carbs, or fats, it does not break down or get absorbed in your body. It serves as food for your gut bacteria.

Though prebiotics can be in supplement form, the most common way to get prebiotics is through the foods we eat. There are many prebiotic foods out there. Here are just a few of them:

- Chicory root—a root with a coffee-like-flavor
- Dandelion greens—great in salads
- Jerusalem artichoke—great cooked or raw
- Garlic—good for flavoring foods
- Onions—good cooked or raw
- Leeks—like onions; good raw or cooked
- Asparagus—good cooked or raw
- Bananas—the greener the better
- Konjac root—also known as elephant yam; a tuber
- Cocoa—a great flavoring or ingredient
- Burdock root—a common Japanese root
- Flaxseeds—a healthy topping to many foods
- Yacon root—like a sweet potato
- Jicama root—good cooked or raw
- Seaweed—common with many Asian dishes[25]

Use as many naturally prebiotic-rich vegetables in your salads or cooked meals as you want. The more it becomes a habit, the better.

RESISTANT STARCHES

Another gut-friendly food is resistant starch. This is the term for carbohydrates that are not digested (they resist it) until they reach the colon, where they ferment and feed the good bacteria in the gut.[26]

Resistant starch "promotes the growth of beneficial bacteria, or probiotics, in the digestive tract; these bacteria then break down the resistant starch into favorable compounds that improve our immune system function and reduce cancer risk."[27]

Common food sources of resistant starches include the following:

- Green plantains
- Green bananas
- Green mangos
- Green papaya
- Sweet potatoes
- Yams

The "green" items above provide particularly healthy carbs, and in their green state they are very low in sugar. According to Dr. Fuhrman, "The healthiest starches are in high fiber, natural foods. These are typically low in absorbable calories, and they give us lots of micronutrients per caloric buck—not just an injection of glucose into our system."[28]

MUSHROOMS AND GARLIC

Dr. Fuhrman points out that there are "several immune-supporting ingredients in mushrooms that empower the body to react quickly and powerfully when we are exposed to disease causing pathogens such as viruses and bacteria. These compounds found in simple mushrooms, have been shown in animal experiments and cell cultures to enhance the activity and function of natural killer T cells."[29]

Garlic has been shown to have antiviral activity. Fresh garlic extract killed each virus tested in one study.[30] I commonly add garlic, onions, and mushrooms to my soups along with chicken, other veggies, and olive oil. Go for the garlic—and buy some sugarless breath mints!

WHAT I EAT

I practice what I preach and eat a plant-based diet with leafy greens, spinach, kale, romaine, arugula, and field green salads with olive oil and lemon on them. For lunch almost every day I enjoy a large salad with lots of veggies and a small amount of grilled chicken breast with grilled onions, plus about four tablespoons of high-phenolic extra-virgin olive oil. It is so tasty, and my wife and I have this almost every day. I have noticed from personal experience that when your gut bacteria shifts, your cravings usually shift away from sugars to healthy foods. Now I actually crave salads with high-phenolic olive oil.

Your body always needs a small to moderate amount of proteins, meaning meats that are organic or grass fed, ideally. I eat lots of soups, as I mentioned before, and lots of berries because they are low in sugar, high in fiber, and bursting with phytonutrients and antioxidants. Colors of the rainbow. I'm a berry nut, and a nut nut as well.

Intermittent fasting is very important. When you fast for sixteen hours and eat in an eight-hour window, it boosts immune function. This basically means skipping breakfast. (For more information, refer to my book *Dr. Colbert's Fasting Zone*.)

Other foods that are fine to round out your diet include the following:

- Coffee and tea (black or green)

- Chocolate (low sugar, 72 percent dark or higher)
- Flours (almond, cassava, coconut, green banana, plantain, arrowroot, sweet potato flours)
- Sweeteners: erythritol, monk fruit sugar, stevia, Just Like Sugar (inulin)
- Seasonings: cocoa powder, capers, saffron, oregano, rosemary, cloves, peppermint, anise, celery seed, sage, spearmint, thyme, basil, curry powder, ginger, cumin, cinnamon

With this mix of ingredients your gut bacteria will thrive and play its proper role in supporting and regulating your immune system. A healthy—and enjoyable—diet will become the most important pillar in your personal health and your preparation for any pandemic. (Refer to appendix A for healthy menus.)

CHAPTER 4

GOOD SLEEP CHARGES THE IMMUNE SYSTEM

I WAS AT HOME recently when suddenly my wife, Mary, screamed, "There's a snake coming through our back door!" I jumped up from the chair where I was sitting and ran into the other room. She was right: a little diamondback rattlesnake was crawling into the house through a hole between the door and the floor! Not having anything else handy, I made an executive decision and threw my hot coffee on the creature to stun it. I'm not sure that did anything more than confuse it for a second, but I was able to grab a nearby chair and pin it to the floor with one of the legs. The snake squirmed and tried to get loose.

"Mary, bring the shovel, quick!" I hollered.

Instead she handed me a nearby broom. The snake was slipping out from under the chair leg and snapping at me by this time. I pinned it against the door with the broom handle, and Mary returned with a shovel. With two tools in hand, I was able to cut off its head.

But for the rest of the day thoughts popped into my mind: "What if that snake had gotten into our house without our knowing it? What might have happened?" I pictured myself walking by that door at night on my way to the fridge and stepping on the snake by accident. "A little snake can kill you," I thought. Before I knew it, I was in a state of worry and concern, and that night it got in the way of my sleep.

When I recognized these thought patterns, I knew I needed to take my own medicine and do what I counsel patients to do: reframe the situation according to God's Word. I prayed, "Thank You, Lord, for protecting me and my wife earlier today. Thank You that You will always protect us from dangers we see and dangers we don't see. Thank You that I can sleep soundly without worrying about this."

I slept soundly, then took practical steps. I had already wedged a small towel to plug the door hole until I had a chance to fashion a more permanent fix. Then I searched the house thoroughly for other unwanted guests of the reptilian kind and found none. I also sealed all cracks and reassured myself that if I got up at night, I would be using a flashlight so I could see where I was walking. We also have motion-sensing lights that illuminate the path so you can see if there's something—like a baby rattlesnake—waiting for you there on the floor.

I haven't had to throw coffee on any more critters since then.

SNAKES ON THE NEWS

Getting my mind back into a state of appreciation and gratitude to God for protecting me and my family solved my minor sleep problem, but the situation reminded me of what happens when a pandemic or any potentially stressful situation hits: the first casualty is usually sleep. During recent outbreaks many people around the globe headed to bed with thoughts of danger filling their minds. They watched the news or read internet headlines right before rolling over and putting their heads on their pillows. They probably had plenty of unsettling "fear" dreams, failed to go into sustained deep sleep, and woke up groggier than ever.

Pandemics present real sleep challenges even to normally peaceful people. We might lie in the dark wondering, "Will I be able to get what I need from the store tomorrow? Is there a possibility that I will catch this virus? What if I already have it? Even worse, what if I unknowingly have shared it with someone who won't physically be able to handle it? And what about our finances? Can we afford this much time off work?"

Even the fact of having to stay indoors can disrupt our sleep. We are forced to stop going to the gym, stop shopping so much, and stop visiting with others. We are forced into a more sedentary, homebound lifestyle, which gets our rhythms and energy level out of whack. We might catch ourselves napping in the middle of the day because there's little else to do. All of this puts deep, restorative sleep at risk—and makes it all the more important to do everything we can to get the good sleep we need.

SLEEP, THE IMMUNITY BOOSTER

Research in recent years shows that sleep affects a wide variety of immune functions, including the number of critically important antigen-fighting cells in our bloodstreams. Specifically, "the proportion of pro-inflammatory and Th1 cytokine...producing T cells [is] profoundly reinforced by sleep." To put that in plain English, it means that two of the most important entities in our immune system reactions are greatly enhanced by sleep. Just as encouraging, the immuno-enhancing effects of sleep are still present over months and years. We can literally accumulate the benefits of strength and "antigenic memory" in our immune systems by having good ongoing sleep habits.[1]

Think of how relatively simple this is. It costs very little. It's something we can do daily, and it's something we can mostly control or support. Getting good sleep by having good "sleep hygiene"—another way of referring to sleep habits—is a choice we can carry out with little more than the will to do it. And it can have transforming effects on every area of our lives.

Poor sleep, to no one's surprise, increases the risk of heart disease. A 2004 study found that women who averaged only five hours of sleep a night were 39 percent more likely to develop heart disease than those who slept eight hours a night.[2] Poor sleep also compromises our immune systems and decreases the number of natural killer cells, resulting in more colds, flu, and other infections. Most everyone knows this by experience.

Though we are wealthy as a nation, we are generally poor in the area of sleep, even in the "good" times. In fact, if prosperity were measured in satisfying and restorative sleep, we might rank near the bottom! It's actually a matter of personal and national defense to get good sleep. Lack of sleep is a silent weakness in our foundation of health, leaving us vulnerable in the face of pandemics, not to mention everyday life.

MY LESSON IN SLEEP DEPRIVATION

I learned this lesson the hard way during medical school and in my early years of medical practice. As a young doctor, I fielded many nighttime calls and messages. I was on call sometimes and only got an hour or two of sleep that night. Over the years as I sacrificed sleep, my energy decreased, I became generally irritable and found it difficult to concentrate.

One thing that concerned me greatly was my forgetfulness. Some mornings Mary would ask me who had called in the middle of the night and awakened us, and I would look at her with uncertainty on my face. I had actually forgotten who had called and whether or not I had phoned in a prescription, and even what the prescription was! Research shows that "just one sleepless night can impair driving performance as much as an alcohol blood level of 0.10 percent," which is higher than the legal limit for driving.[3] I was living that statistic.

I knew things were way off course with my health when I became so fatigued that I began putting my car in park when I stopped at a red light because I feared I would fall asleep at the light. The next "alarms" to go off were in my immune system as I suffered from recurrent colds and sinus infections. I also developed irritable bowel syndrome with abdominal bloating, abdominal pains, and bouts of diarrhea. As my lack of sleep continued, the alarms kept ringing, and I eventually developed psoriasis and chronic fatigue. One morning I awakened with intense itching and a rash on my legs that would not go away though I applied hydrocortisone cream to it. Rather, it spread across my body. Of course, I didn't ascribe it to my sleep-deprived state. Rather, I thought I might have contracted scabies from a patient I had seen recently!

Financial debt from opening up a solo private practice while paying off medical-school loans also weighed heavily on my emotions. Like many physicians I also feared potential lawsuits and found the rising costs of malpractice insurance to be a staggering financial burden. The more I suffered from infections and irritable bowel syndrome, the more fatigue I felt and the weaker my immune system became. I had reached a dead end in my health. Here I was a medical doctor, but I was sick—I was literally stewing in my own juices and saw no way out of my predicament.

I realize now that I had accumulated a huge sleep debt and had lost the vitality, energy, and mental clarity that only sleep can provide. My body and mind needed a certain amount of sleep per night in order to function at their best, and I was withholding that sleep. My body, mind, and emotions couldn't help but react with various problems.

The road back to health began when I discovered how important it is to get restorative sleep. People who sleep nine hours a night instead of seven hours have greater than normal "natural killer cell" activity. Most adults need seven to nine hours of sleep a night without interruption. Infants need more—about twelve to fifteen hours a day. A five-year-old needs ten to thirteen hours a day.[4] Most people find that eight hours is perfect.

I learned that the REM stage of sleep and the phases of deep sleep are by far the most important stages of sleep. It is deep, restorative, and refreshing. That's why it's critically important to get uninterrupted, peaceful sleep for the first three sleep cycles, which get us to the much-needed REM stage and the deep sleep, where the overnight repair and rejuvenation work is done.

SLEEP APNEA IS A VERY REAL PROBLEM

Many people over fifty, especially if they are obese, have undiagnosed sleep apnea and are not getting restorative sleep. As a result, their immune systems are faltering. You need to be checked for sleep apnea if your spouse reports that you stop breathing for a few seconds while sleeping or gasp for air, you snore loudly, you awaken with a dry mouth or morning hoarseness, or you experience excessive daytime sleepiness.[5]

Discovering the value of sleep changed my patients' lives as well. I began to recognize when sleep deprivation was the source of their diseases and problems, and I developed and prescribed keys for getting good sleep, which is foundational to a robust immune response.

25 SLEEP HYGIENE HABITS

Here are twenty-five immune-boosting sleep hygiene habits that will help you to fall asleep, and stay asleep, even in times of global trouble.

1. The most important sleep hygiene tip is to establish a regular bedtime. Stick to the schedule on weekends and even during vacations. Do not be haphazard about it, but based on your work schedule, set aside eight hours for sleep and a time to be in bed. For myself, I choose to be in bed between 10:00 and 10:30 p.m.

2. Use your bed only for sleep and sexual relations. Do not use your bed for reading, watching TV, snacking, working—or worrying!

3. Avoid naps after 3:00 p.m. If you take one earlier in the day, make sure it is not longer than twenty to thirty minutes.

4. Exercise before dinner, but not too close to bedtime. Engage in some sort of aerobic exercise, such as brisk walking in the afternoon or early evening. Daily exercise is one of the best ways to improve the quality of your sleep because it helps you fall asleep faster and sleep longer. People who exercise spend a greater amount of time in stage three and four sleep.

   But don't go overboard and rev up your body with exercise within three hours of bedtime. It heats up your body and raises the stress hormones. Not long ago I took a sauna too close to bedtime and got so hot that I couldn't sleep well. What a mistake! Exercise is good, but do it earlier in the day.

5. Avoid caffeine in the late afternoon and evening. Some people can handle caffeine; others can't. If you fall in the latter category, then do yourself a favor and quit drinking or eating caffeinated products by noon.

6. Avoid excessive fluids in the late evening and especially before bedtime. Getting up to use the bathroom obviously interrupts sleep.

7. Eat normal portion sizes of a well-balanced meal at dinnertime around three to four hours before bedtime as well as a light bedtime snack. Do not go to bed hungry, and do not eat a large meal prior to bedtime. A snack that is correctly balanced with proteins, carbohydrates, and fats will help stabilize blood sugar through the nighttime hours.

8. Take a warm bath one to two hours before bedtime, and consider adding lavender oil if desired in order to help you relax.

9. Keep your bedroom cool and well ventilated.

10. Clean clutter out of the bedroom, and remove computers, fax machines, paperwork, and anything that reminds you of work.

11. Purchase a comfortable mattress, pillow, and linens. You spend roughly one-third of your life in bed, so treat your bed as your most important piece of furniture. This may be the one area where you need to financially splurge!

12. Thirty minutes before going to bed, start to wind down by listening to soothing music, reading the Bible or another good book, or being intimate with your spouse.

13. Put dimmer switches on your lights and dim them a few hours prior to bedtime. As the sun goes down, your body will relax naturally. Before electricity was developed, almost everyone went to bed when it was dark and awakened whenever it was light outside. Now, however, with the help of bright lights, TVs, computer screens, and more, many have confused their brains into thinking that it is daytime when in reality it is the middle of the night. Also, nightclubs, late-night shopping and dining, late-night movies, the internet,

shift work, and artificial lighting have disrupted many
people's circadian rhythm.

You are designed hormonally to stay in sync with
the cycles of nature. When the light fades, the hormone melatonin is released into your bloodstream,
making you sleepy. Flow with the passage of day
and night—don't fight them.

14. Try exchanging foot, neck and shoulder, back, or scalp
massages with your spouse.

15. Relax your mind and body before bedtime by gentle
stretching, relaxation exercises, or using an aroma-
therapy candle or oil.

16. Make sure your bedroom is completely dark. Remove
all nightlights, and cover your alarm clock and phone
light with a hand towel. Put black electrical tape or
sticky notepads over tiny lights on your alarm system,
TV, DVD, satellite, stereo, or any other lights that are
visible. Consider purchasing blackout curtains.

17. Block out noise by using earplugs, double-paning
your windows, or using heavy drapes. I personally use
a sound generator that plays white noise. Or you can
simply use a fan.

18. Try a lullaby CD or a CD that has sounds of nature.

19. Keep pets out of your bedroom. Pets may snore,
pounce on you, growl, howl, bark, or whine. They can
also trigger allergies in many patients.

20. Avoid watching heart-pounding movies, sporting
events, or late-night news—especially when the world
is gripped by a crisis such as a pandemic. Instead
watch something funny or lighthearted before bedtime—or, even better, don't watch TV in the bedroom
at all. Much of what is on TV gets our hearts and
minds moving faster. Even "good" stress can raise our

cortisol levels, which disrupts the neurotransmitter balance in the brain, causing you to be more irritable and prone to anxiety and insomnia. Good sleep helps to reduce cortisol levels. Do your mind a favor and unplug from the news and entertainment world before heading to bed.

21. Good sleep is something to tackle with your husband or wife. If he or she is up at night, it disrupts your sleep patterns. Sleeping in separate rooms is not ideal. If he or she is upset or energized by watching something too late, or being anxious about what's happening in the world, this offers a great opportunity to come into unity, being of one mind in peace and confidence in the Lord.

    When lying in bed, you and your spouse may try telling or reading funny jokes to one another. Couples who laugh together and pray together generally stay together.

22. Together and individually meditate on Scripture, and do not let your mind worry or wander. I meditate on the Lord's Prayer in Matthew 6:9–13. I also meditate on Psalm 23, Psalm 91, 1 Corinthians 13:4–8, Psalm 127:2, and Ephesians 6:10–18. Memorize these scriptures and meditate on them over and over.

    This helps you to corral your thoughts. As the evening goes on and your mind wanders over the events of the day, don't let anxiety derail you from your goal. Switch from the "worry" channel to the "appreciation and praise" channel. Make a list of things for which you are thankful, and then dwell on those instead.

23. After you lie down to go to sleep, if you are not asleep in twenty minutes, simply get up, go into another room, and read and relax in dim light until you feel sleepy. Then return to bed.

24. If your spouse awakens you with snoring or unusual movements, simply move to the guest bedroom for the time being.

25. Try to wake up at the same time each day.

HELP WITH SLEEP

When people have trouble sleeping anyway, there are some natural ways to encourage the process. Two supplements in particular can be taken orally, and they can help.

Melatonin

Melatonin is a hormone produced by a small gland, called the pineal gland, in the brain. Melatonin helps to regulate sleep and wake cycles. Usually melatonin begins to rise in the evening and remains high for most of the night and then decreases in the early morning. Melatonin production is affected by light. As a person ages, melatonin levels decline. Older adults typically produce very small amounts of melatonin or none at all. Studies suggest that melatonin induces sleep without suppressing REM or dream sleep, whereas most sleep meds suppress REM sleep.[6] Start with 1 mg of melatonin at bedtime and increase to 3–5 mg if needed. Some people need even higher doses.

L-tryptophan and 5-HTP (5-hydroxytryptophan)

Both L-tryptophan and its metabolite 5-HTP are used to increase serotonin levels in the brain. Serotonin is a neurotransmitter in the brain that promotes restful sleep and well-being. I commonly place patients with insomnia on melatonin and the amino acid L-tryptophan or 5-HTP. L-tryptophan improves sleep normalcy and increases stage three sleep. It has also been shown to improve obstructive sleep apnea in many patients. I usually recommend 5-HTP 150–200 mg at bedtime.

No matter what happens in the world, we have a sure promise from the Word of God that "He gives His beloved sleep" (Ps. 127:2). While the Bible promises us a good night's sleep, we have to do our part in order to obtain it. Meditate on God's Word and not on the problems swirling around us. Isaiah 26:3 says, "You will keep him in perfect peace, whose mind is stayed on You."

If people built strong foundations in these two areas—a healthy diet and good sleep—they would be less likely to get viruses, and less likely for illnesses to turn into something serious. Diet and sleep are the cornerstones of a powerful, resistant immune system. But there is much more we can do to shield ourselves from sweeping pandemics. For more information on sleep, refer to my books *The New Bible Cure for Sleep Disorders* and *The Ultimate Sleep Guide*.

CHAPTER 5

PEACE, JOY, AND LAUGHTER CHARGE THE IMMUNE SYSTEM AND DEFEAT STRESS

THERE'S A TYPE of warfare called psychological operations—psyops, for short—which is all about defeating the enemy in his own head. During wartime each side churns out propaganda designed to encourage their side and discourage the other side. This propaganda takes the form of radio broadcasts, movies, newspaper and magazine articles, and much more. In wars as early as the nineteenth century, airplanes or even balloons dropped leaflets on an opponent's territory declaring that his army will never win, and giving helpful instructions for how to surrender. Radio broadcasts into foreign countries announced the imminent triumph of one army over another, with "news" tailored to make the listening audience feel demoralized and defeated already. These psychological efforts, which have worked very effectively for thousands of years in wartime, are about winning the battle of the mind. Once a nation has lost the war in its head, it is as good as defeated.

This is a good picture of what happens in people's minds during pandemics. They become psyops battlegrounds—and sometimes our own worst enemy is right between our ears. When we believe the worst news, and exclude or discount good news, and when we take our own anxious thoughts as facts rather than mere emotions, we wave the white flag in the face of the invader. We literally weaken our immune response at the time we need it most.

Winning the battle against pandemics has a lot to do with this battle in our minds. This chapter is about confidently gaining victory by filling our minds with peace, joy, and certainty—attitudes that boost the immune system and lead to strength, optimism, and sure triumph over any type of invader.

THE ENEMY IN YOUR HEAD

Chronic stress never did anybody any good, least of all in critical situations. Chronic stressors are associated with the suppression of both cellular and humoral immune responses.[1]

Chronic stress also contributes to the activation of latent viruses, meaning that the viruses your system had neutralized suddenly gain the upper hand and begin fighting with fresh vigor.[2]

- According to a Mayo Clinic study of people with heart disease, psychological stress was a strong predictor of future cardiac events.[3]

- Most worrisome of all during any kind of contagious pandemic is how stress hammers away at our immune response. Dr. Hans Selye showed that rats exposed to chronic stress developed shrunken thymus glands.[4] Chronic stress in humans has also been associated with atrophy or shrinking of the thymus gland, as well as decreased function of the thymus gland. We know from looking at our immune systems that the thymus gland is perhaps the most important immune organ we have. Anything that shrinks or weakens it damages our bodies and resistance to flus, bacteria, and other antigens.

- In fact, elevated cortisol levels are associated with as much as a 50 percent reduction of natural killer cells that destroy cancer cells, bacteria, and viruses.[5] Elevated cortisol levels increase a person's susceptibility for developing recurrent infections. Students in one study were shown to be more prone to catch a cold, develop cold sores, or get infections when stressed during final-exam week.[6]

Now imagine that final-exam week lasting for months, and the entire world taking the finals at the same time. That's essentially the atmosphere that pandemics create—global, group stress from which there seems to be no escape. Pandemics place another layer of stress on top of the stress modern life already brings. Shopping and community life are disrupted. Some critical items are scarce. Jobs are lost or put on hold. People are forced to stay home, often with other family members whose company they would enjoy more if they weren't together twenty-four hours a day. All conversations turn to the present pandemic and how people are reacting. News of someone being affected and even dying reaches our ears via friends and social media.

Pandemics have every potential to produce stress responses around the clock.

The good news is that bad stress is based not on actual events but on our reactions to our perceptions—and our reactions are within our control. It all comes down to how we choose to perceive and think. Dr. David Burns, a renowned psychiatrist and author of *Feeling Good*, identified ten distortional thought processes[7] I like to expand upon as a basis for defeating stress and creating a beautiful, strong atmosphere of peace and joy within our own souls, in our homes, and in our communities. We will identify the negative pattern and remove its power by replacing it with a better way of thinking.

I believe that replacing stress with peace and joy is the third-most powerful way to protect against pandemics. Let's go to the front lines of our minds and win the battle.

TEN DISTORTIONAL THOUGHT PATTERNS

1. "What if" thinking

During a pandemic or outbreak you probably have heard people say things like, "What if I get this virus?" "What if I lose my job?" "What if someone I love dies of this?" Those thoughts may even find their way inside your own mind. But "what if" thinking almost always leads to anxiety and fear. As believers we have a sure future, we are told in God's Word. We don't live in a "what if" reality but rather a "God said" reality. God's Word says that He always causes us to triumph, that He will take care of all of our needs, that He will never fail to provide for us and protect us. As you read these scriptural promises, I'm sure you can already feel the confidence rising up inside of you.

During times of global pressure we must speak specifically about what is taking place around us from a perspective of faith. We can actually turn the what-ifs into positives! "What if this crisis produces good results in families, health care responses, and other ways we don't even see yet?" "What if not nearly as many people are affected as the estimates say?" "What if I get a better job or more opportunities as a result of this?"

If you're going to get stuck in "what if" thinking, aim it in a positive direction!

2. Catastrophizing

I call this kind of thinking "awfulizing" because the mind actually magnifies unpleasant events and transforms them into something more awful or horrible than they really are. If you want an example of awfulizing, just watch the news. News stations make their money by awfulizing virtually everything—especially outbreaks and pandemics.

But awfulizing can take place in every arena of life. You may stand in line to buy toilet paper, only to have it run out before you get to the rack. Someone who "awfulizes" situations will see this as a sure sign that they will never get the supplies they need. They will go home depressed and defeated—and probably turn on the news and make themselves feel even worse!

Years ago I seemed to always be standing in the shortest line at the grocery store, only to have it turn into the longest line! Someone ahead of me would have a credit card declined, the clerk would need a price check on an item, the cash register would run out of tape, or the manager would need to approve a check. I would awfulize the situation and become very frustrated. All I was doing was making the consequences seem much greater than they were. I was only delayed by a few minutes, but I could make myself feel like that one delay had thrown off my entire week.

At some point I wised up to the battle in my head and decided to quit awfulizing those moments and instead reframe them. Instead of seeing the delay in terms of frustration, I chose to see it as an opportunity for a relaxation break—a time to practice a couple of deep-breathing exercises along with some posture-related exercises or to check my emails or text messages. The delayed lines became not only beneficial to me but also even pleasurable.

I "awesomized" those moments!

In pandemics, and really in every arena of life at all times, each one of us can awesomize rather than awfulize our circumstances.

3. Habitually expecting the worst outcome

When the COVID-19 pandemic swept the world, some people responded by saying, "I've been waiting for this thing to hit." It's like they were expecting to get it! Their faith was in Murphy's Law, which states that anything that *can* go wrong *will* go wrong. People tend to personalize that and think, "If something bad is going to happen, it will probably happen to me."

This is such a dangerous habit. All thoughts can become self-fulfilling prophecies. Galatians 6:7 says, "Do not be deceived, God is not mocked; for whatever a man sows, that he will also reap." In other words, if you plant worst-case-scenario thoughts, you will eventually reap a worst-case-scenario harvest. If you think, "Well, I've been waiting for that deadly flu or bacteria to come, and now it's here," you are lowering your shields to allow it in. Willingly you go along because you think it's inevitable. Next thing you know, you're in a hospital on a ventilator saying, "See? I told you so."

There's an old joke that makes the point. For years a wife would tell her husband when they were lying in bed, "Harvey, there's a burglar downstairs. Go down and see." For fifty years there never was a burglar. Finally one night, Harvey went downstairs yet again at his wife's request, and there in the kitchen stood an actual burglar. "Can you wait here?" Harvey said to the man. "My wife has been waiting for you for fifty years, and I want her to finally meet you."

Instead of expecting the worst possible outcome, begin to expect something good to happen to you. Use those "what if" scenarios like a weapon against Murphy's Law. Dethrone that terrible "law" and enthrone the law of Christ in your life! It works.

4. Leaping to conclusions

I call these people "grim leapers." They mistakenly believe that they know what another person is thinking without having any facts to support it. They repeatedly and habitually make negative assumptions that fuel their anxiety.

For example, someone declines your invitation to dinner during a pandemic, and you think they don't value you anymore, when in fact they feel run-down and don't want to expose you to anything harmful. Or their motivation may not even be related to the pandemic. It's far too easy to misread someone's motivations and to read our own fears into their actions.

Let's leap to good conclusions and give people the benefit of our trust and love.

5. Black-and-white thinking

People who suffer from this thought pattern view circumstances in black and white, with no shades of gray. They are perfectionists who see their work as either flawless or worthless. All news is either amazing or terrible. There is no in between.

At a deeper level such people tend to be perfectionists. They gain a false sense of control by thinking, "If I control everything in my environment, I and my family will be protected. But if I fail at one little thing, our protection is compromised."

This kind of all-or-nothing perspective is built to fail, and it causes a constantly elevated level of stress as "perfection" is attempted to be maintained.

The good news is that God never expects us to attain perfection. The Bible even promises that righteous people will fall many times, but each time they will get up and press on. That's the lifestyle of the believer: rejecting prideful perfectionism for humble but relentless pursuit of God.

6. Unenforceable rules

This person has a rigid set of rules about what *should*, *must*, or *ought to* be done, and tries to put people and events into a little box. The person's expectations are unrealistic because nobody has control over circumstances or other people. The more unrealistic and unenforceable the rules are, the greater this person's disappointment.

During pandemics people's rules get firmer and more numerous. Their expectations go well beyond realistic. You might think, "Why doesn't everyone wear masks and stop going in public unless they absolutely must?" Or you might think, "Why can't people chill out and be a little more friendly? We're all going through this together. A simple 'hello' wouldn't hurt." Every one of us lives by certain rules, but when we bring our set of expectations to interactions with others, we find that people rarely meet them all. In fact, many expectations are in direct opposition to each other, so it is impossible to fulfill everyone's "rules."

The healthy person knows that the only *should* statement we need to make is "I should do everything I can to give love and mercy, especially during this time when people's emotions are so frayed." The good news is that when you give love and mercy instead of insisting that people follow your unenforceable rules, you will receive love and mercy in return.

That's a recipe for a more relaxed and healthier community.

7. Labeling

Pandemics can bring out the worst instincts to label and denigrate other people. Some label others as "fear-mongers" for being concerned about public health, while others accuse those who are not openly worried of being careless and cavalier with their lives and the lives of others. Insults start piling up: "Ignorant." "Unscientific." "Foolhardy." "Insensitive." "Controlling." These and many other unkind words get thrown around during a time of health crisis.

All degrading words separate and divide, leaving each of us

weaker than before. Labels destroy the very sense of love and belonging we need to have during times of heightened challenge.

Loving others sincerely from our hearts is the healthiest thing we can do (Rom. 12). Paul described believers are being like a human body; every part needs every other part. It does no good to emphasize the differences and delegitimize each other. Let's respect and learn from the different perspectives and values each of us brings to the table. If you have to label someone, make it a positive label!

8. Negative filter

You've met this person: he or she discounts or discredits all positive information. You might say, "It looks like the rate of infection is lower than they previously thought," and he will say, "Yes, but did you hear about the new cruise ship that's been infected?" People like this have a "talent" for retaining all bad information while allowing anything good to slip away. They find the gray lining in every silver cloud.

Make sure you're not one of these people. Replace your filter so you highlight the good stuff and not the bad.

9. Emotional reasoning

This person treats feelings as facts. Anxiety becomes a firm reality. Perceived danger becomes actual, not just an imagination.

Because our emotions are drawn to rise and fall with news cycles and a myriad of other factors, it pays during pandemics to distinguish emotions from facts. When we do, we remove the steering wheel of our minds from the grip of our emotions.

10. The blame game

In crisis moments the temptation is often to blame others or God for what is happening. People feel they are victims of unfair circumstances, and they want to assign blame for everything bad that happens to them. During a recent pandemic I heard people say things like, "It's that other country's fault. They should have been more transparent and up-front with the rest of us."

And, "Our own leaders failed us. They should have acted quicker."

And, "Our leaders acted too quickly and did more harm than good. They turned America into a police state for a while."

There are serious issues to discuss regarding national and personal responses to extreme health crises, but those discussions never move forward on the wings of blame. Indeed, even during non-crisis times I have been amazed at how many of my patients come into my office with a complaining, whining, critical attitude. When I prescribe "the speaking of stress-relieving words" to my patients—that is, the speaking of positive, life-affirming words and phrases—their conditions often improve dramatically.

To complain is to lower your walls of immunity. In the past few years there has been considerable research on living with a mindset of gratitude. Researchers have found that gratitude and the positive emotions it fosters can help you create a higher income, create superior work outcomes, experience a longer and better marriage, have more friends, have stronger social supports, have more energy, enjoy better overall physical health, develop a stronger immune system, have better cardiovascular health, lower your stress levels, and enjoy a longer life (up to ten years longer in one study).[8]

That's a bunch of benefits!

Our words have tremendous power to cause or relieve stress in our own lives. Remember that the war between fear and peace takes place primarily in our heads first. Whether we say them or just think them, the words we "speak" always reach their most eager audience—ourselves. Wise King Solomon wrote that "Death and life are in the power of the tongue, and those who love it will eat its fruit" (Prov. 18:21). Notice that we eat the fruit of our own words. When we speak carelessly or critically, we can cause tremendous stress to dominate our own minds. Nothing we say goes unnoticed by God or by our own ears. Everything we say promotes either life or death.

Our attitudes and words spill over to affect others. Proverbs 25:11 says a word fitly spoken is like apples of gold in settings of silver. That a cheerful word is like a kiss on the lips, and brings light to someone's face. How would you characterize your own speech? Do you choose positive, encouraging, comforting, kind, gentle, caring words? Be honest with yourself right now: What kinds of conversations have you initiated or participated in during times of crisis and pandemic? Did they foster a worrisome outlook, or a confident, joyful one?

Now ask the same questions about your social media posts and texts. What message have you been sending to people around you? Do you share fear-inducing headlines and stories? Conspiracy-oriented stuff? How are you contributing to a faith-filled atmosphere in your social circle and the world around you?

For some people the response to those questions is likely to be, "Ouch."

LIVING IN RHYTHM WITH LIFE

Physicians can measure the function of the autonomic nervous system in several ways. One way is by what has come to be called "heart rate variability," the measure of beat-to-beat changes in the heart rate as it speeds up and slows down in different patterns. Emotions and attitudes can especially influence heartbeat changes.

- Appreciation, joy, and love create a coherent spectrum on the heart rate variability EKG tracing. These emotions and attitudes enable a person to enter into a healthy state called *entrainment*. When a person has entered into entrainment, the sympathetic nervous system and the parasympathetic nervous system are fully synchronized or balanced. This allows a person to enjoy just the right amount of stimulation and the right amount of relaxation. If a person consciously chooses to focus on things that evoke a sense of appreciation or gratitude, the nervous system comes back into balance, and all systems of the body—the brain included—function in greater harmony.[9]

- But toxic emotions such as frustration, bitterness, anger, resentment, and anxiety can cause an incoherent heart rate variability spectrum. Why? Because they create imbalance in the sympathetic and parasympathetic nervous systems, and as a result they are not fully synchronized. The Institute of HeartMath has also found that compassion and kindness add energy to a physical body. According to the Institute, these core heart feelings increase synchronization and coherence in the heart rhythm patterns, and these in turn decrease stress.[10]

The battle in our heads comes down to a choice: Fear or Peace? Proverbs assures us that the peaceful mind is the powerful, victorious mind. Jesus said, "My peace I give to you.... Take heart, for I have overcome the world." (See John 16:33 and 14:27.) Peace is not passive acceptance of whatever "hand you are dealt." Peace is a posture of power and victory. Peace overcomes. It actively guards our hearts and minds in Christ Jesus.

During pandemics and other potentially stressful times, choose to go in the opposite direction from fear. Video call some family members for dinner. Watch funny and wholesome shows or movies. Ratchet down expectations on those around you. I recommend ten belly laughs a day. King Solomon wrote, "A cheerful heart is good medicine" (Prov. 17:22, NIV). He must have observed how cheerfulness affected the health of lives around him. I tell my patients that laughter is as powerful as a drug, very inexpensive, and has absolutely no side effects. Paul described the kingdom of heaven as "righteousness and peace and joy in the Holy Spirit" (Rom. 14:17).

Then practice gratitude. Be thankful you don't have the virus, that you have a place to live, that you have basic supplies. In the recent COVID-19 pandemic I found myself thanking God for toilet paper, hand sanitizer, and paper towels! I never thought I'd pray that kind of prayer, but it came from my heart. Gratitude reframes your whole situation. I am thankful that my children and grandkids stayed safe and got to enjoy school at home for a period of time. I am grateful for how our family grew together by being home more, sharing meals, cooking together, and enjoying wholesome entertainment together.

Then give the gift of mercy, because pandemics produce lots of stressed-out people. On the highways or in line at the store, be courteous and gracious. Don't fight for position or products but try to serve others with your attitude, your approach to shopping, and the atmosphere you carry with you. All of this will help us to win the battle of the mind. For more information on overcoming stress, refer to my book *Stress Less*.

War historians speak of the tide of war turning. Most often this occurs when something happens to make one side believe they are going to win the war. Their morale shoots sky-high, while the morale of the other side plummets. These are decisive moments in war and in human history—and they are mostly the result of what both sides think about what happened.

Winston Churchill is considered one of the greatest statesmen of the twentieth century because when things looked darkest for Great Britain—when they could have easily lost the war in their heads—he declared, "We shall never surrender."[11] He made his country believe they could defeat what appeared to be a much stronger opponent. And they did.

You can too.

CHAPTER 6

EXERCISE CHARGES THE IMMUNE SYSTEM

WHEN COVID-19 HIT, I found myself with more extra time than I'd had in years, mainly because I couldn't really do very many in-person visits with patients until the pandemic had passed since most of my patients are from out of state or out of the country and couldn't fly in. One of my first actions was to get Mary's and my bicycles out of the garage and pump their tires up. If we couldn't do much else, at least we were going to enjoy the scenery!

We already have a small workout gym at our home, so the pandemic didn't change our regular workouts, but when life slows down and you're stuck at home for weeks, you start looking for other things to do. I had purchased these electric bikes a couple of years ago, which were just about the coolest things I'd ever seen on two wheels. They could be pedaled like an ordinary bike, or you could flip a switch and an electric motor would supplement your pedaling. Wow! Those things could take off—up to twenty-five miles per hour. It was invigorating.

Mary and I wanted to be able to ride together with each of us doing our preferred level of intensity. When I chose to really exert myself, she could switch on the motor and keep up with me—and usually pass me! After a good heart-pumping time I would click on my motor and cruise along with her.

Those rides were some of the most enjoyable of our lives. Beyond the workout it gave us, we got to experience the fresh air and sunshine, the wind blowing, and the views we encountered along the way. I wouldn't trade those days for anything.

My observation, and what I hear from others as well, is that during COVID-19, many people used their free time to exercise more. Greenbelts were full of walking and jogging people, living rooms were turned into workout rooms with online instructors, and women did dance aerobics in their kitchens while the guys dusted off the weights in the garage. That pandemic may have produced one of the healthiest time periods in American history! Many stores sold out of workout equipment, dumbbells, and barbells.

What many people probably didn't realize was that exercise and an active lifestyle are about more than feeling good and looking good; exercise powerfully supports our immune systems and works against the pandemic! Exercise is like maintaining a strong fighting force. In peacetime, when there is no pandemic or outbreak, it's like soldiers marching up and down an empty field at an army base, or sailors conducting maneuvers on a ship in the ocean. Exercise makes our bodies vibrant and ready to repel any incoming attack. It puts our bodies in an efficient position to overcome pandemics.

America's exercise response to the COVID-19 pandemic was just right.

THE SCIENCE

The findings of researchers at the University of Virginia strongly suggest that exercising regularly can reduce the risk of acute respiratory distress syndrome (ARDS), which is a major cause of death in patients with the COVID-19 virus.[1]

Beyond that, study after study shows that regular exercise is a key to good health, and good health is key to our body's preparation for attacks. As one expert puts it, "Regular exercise can enhance vaccination responses, increase T-cells and boost the function of the natural killer cells in the immune system. Exercise also lowers levels of the inflammatory cytokines that cause the 'inflamm-ageing' that is thought to play a role in conditions including cardiovascular disease; type 2 diabetes; Alzheimer's disease; osteoporosis and some cancers."[2]

One study looked at aerobic exercise as a means of treating clinical depression. An aerobic exercise program was compared to standard medication in a group of older adult patients. The experiment lasted sixteen weeks. Medication relieved symptoms of depression more rapidly at the outset, but aerobic exercise was shown to be equally effective to medication over the course of the four-month study. Since some medications for depression have adverse effects or cease to be as effective with prolonged use, this was an important finding—aerobic exercise may be a very viable long-term therapy.[3]

Regular exercise decreases the stress hormone cortisol. It boosts endorphins, the morphine-like compounds that elevate your mood, enable you to sleep better, and decrease muscle tension. Even moderate aerobic exercise has a calming effect on the body and diminishes the response to stress for up to four hours after the exercise session.

One way that exercise supports immunity is by maintaining a healthy lymphatic system. The lymphatic system is a major microbe crime-fighter and cellular garbage collector in the body. It removes toxins and cellular waste, and it "keeps the peace" by rounding up bacteria, viruses, and other bad guys, bringing them to the lymph nodes where they are killed by white blood cells. Lymphatic fluid is so important that your body contains about three times more lymph than blood. The lymphatic fluid moves around via very small vessels, which usually run alongside small veins and arteries.

But the lymphatic system has no "heart" or pumping mechanism. Rather, lymphatic fluid is circulated by muscle contractions, not by your heartbeat. When you don't move, the lymphatic system becomes sluggish. Aerobic exercise can triple the rate of lymphatic flow. That means the lymphatic system—part of your in-house defense force—does a much better job protecting your body from attack when you are active and moving.

The same can be said for a strong cardiovascular system.

Everything works better when our blood is flowing freely through our vessels and our hearts are beating strongly and consistently. This includes the humoral immune agents—those that travel in the bloodstream—which move about more easily and work more efficiently when our blood flow is good.

All kinds of studies show that moderate, regular exercise is perhaps the single most important deterrent of heart-related problems. When pandemics come, they often attack those with existing physical problems, commonly things like heart disease, lung disease, and cancer. Aerobic exercise reduces coronary risk factors. It helps lower blood pressure, lowers blood triglyceride levels (fats), lowers the bad (LDL) cholesterol, raises the good (HDL) cholesterol, and may prevent blood clots. In a study where researchers monitored over 84,000 nurses for fourteen years, the nurses who exercised regularly had a 41 percent lower risk of both heart attack and stroke when compared to sedentary women.[4]

All of this is critical to how our bodies handle viral and bacterial invaders. Are your heart and lungs strong? Is your lymphatic system getting enough movement? If not, now is the time to start—don't wait until the next pandemic strikes.

How to Exercise Well

Nobody has to go to the gym to work out. In fact, I strongly counsel you not to go to a gym during a potential outbreak! Many gyms closed down anyway during COVID-19. A gym is not a good place to be when infectious agents are in the air—and on towels, walls, exercise bikes, benches, weights, and more. No amount of cleaning and wiping down can keep up with a persistent virus waiting to meet its next host.

My top recommendation for exercise is virtually free—unless you count the cost of walking shoes. Brisk walking is the best low-impact aerobic exercise I know of. It supplies you three times the normal amount of oxygen you would otherwise get. Make sure to walk slow enough so that you can talk, but fast enough so that you can't sing. Window-shopping doesn't count. Keep a steady pace without stopping.

There are times to do more intense exercises like running or working out on elliptical machines, exercise bikes, and treadmills. When you do, aim for your specific target heart rate during exercise. This can be figured by subtracting your age from 220, multiplying that by .6 (60 percent), and then multiplying the original number again times .8 (80 percent). The range between the two numbers is your target heart rate range. For example, if you are forty years old:

220 - 40 = 180; 180 x .6 = 108 low target;
180 x .8 = 144 high target

In this example, the target heart rate is between 108 and 144 beats per minute. If you push much higher than your target heart rate, you are probably stressing your body too much and may be doing more harm than good. If you have not been exercising, initially aim for the lower target heart rate number and listen to your body.

I also counsel anyone over age thirty to exercise with weights or calisthenics to keep their muscles and bones strong. Low-intensity workouts are not harmful. When possible, have a certified trainer teach you safe ways to do exercises on the eight to ten different muscle groups in your chest, back, shoulders, arms, abdomen, upper and lower back, and legs and calves. It's important to maintain proper form and work your full range of motion. Ideally you should work out with weights three days per week with a day between workouts.

Here are some other tips to keep you moving and strengthening your body:

- *Build exercise into your schedule.* The greatest benefits of aerobic exercise tend to occur if a person exercises early in the morning. However, the time a person does aerobic exercise is not nearly as important as the frequency and duration of the exercise. You should do aerobic exercises three to five times a week for twenty to thirty minutes each time. Schedule it like an important doctor's appointment.

- *Choose an exercise you enjoy.* The best exercise is the one you'll do. If you do not enjoy the exercise activity you are doing, chances are you will not stick with it. Find an exercise or activity that you do enjoy, and set a reasonable goal; instead of exercising five to seven days a week, try exercising every other day or three times a week. Have a day in between to rest. Start out walking only five or ten minutes a day, and gradually increase the time as well as the pace.

- *Have an exercise partner.* Partners keep you accountable to do the exercise and should make the exercise time more enjoyable.

- *Choose a location you enjoy.* Walk in parks, in the mountains, on the beach, or near a lake. Make exercise a complete sensory experience, like Mary and I do on our bike rides. Of course, during pandemics, malls and hiking trails can be closed, depending on where you live, so choose the wise alternative. Simply walking around a neighbor-hood or open space is great.

- *Change it up.* Change your routine, either by loca-tion, time of day, or by the exercise you do. Make it fun.

- *Do occupational/transportation exercises.* Seize every opportunity to increase your activity level. Park at the far end of the parking lot and walk to the store. Use stairs when you can.

DON'T OVERDO IT

One of my concerns for people during COVID-19 was that some seemed to jump into large amounts of exercise because they had little else to do. This can lead to injury because they demand things of their bodies that their bodies are not prepared to do. Ease into a new routine. Just because you have more time and the desire to get a healthier immune system doesn't mean you can sprint your way to success. Slow and steady wins the race, giving you long-term health that can be sustained in and out of times of crisis and prevents injury or a heart attack.

Researchers have found that extremes of exercise—usually per-formed by endurance athletes—can actually elevate cortisol levels. Overtraining can suppress the immune system and interfere with emotions and mental function.

For years I pushed my body very hard, until I had a heat stroke and almost died. I had not allowed my body to stop when it needed to stop. Now, older and wiser, I have slowed my pace, and I listen to what my body is saying.

I have talked at length with many highly trained athletes, including marathon runners and professional athletes, who are compulsive exercise enthusiasts. The downside of compulsive exercise is that many of these people suffer from constant muscle soreness from overtraining, and chronic fatigue. By contrast I recommend low-intensity workouts and moderation in physical exertion, because the pressure associated with excessive exercise can undo the very thing you are trying to accomplish.

SAUNA THERAPY

Another good way to prepare your body physically for pandemic challenges is to heat it up through sauna therapy, especially in an infrared sauna. Like exercise, this charges the immune system. One study of Finnish sauna sessions reported that they "stimulate the immune system" and that "hot-cold bathing reduces susceptibility to colds and prevents infections in healthy subjects." In this study, "The lymphocyte count...rose significantly in the group of trained men. One of the subpopulations of lymphocytes is natural killer lymphocytes (NK). Another study found an increase in NK count as a response to the exposure to thermal stress."[5]

I spend thirty minutes in an infrared sauna that is between 130 and 150 degrees, usually right after an aerobic workout, and drink plenty of alkaline water, which I recommend for its detoxifying and immune boosting benefits.

When exercise, diet, and sleep are aligned properly it creates the most invigorating, immune-healthy lifestyle. Each one supports the other. There is a sense of balance and fulfillment. But there are other things you can do to supplement your body's response in times of global health crises. Let's continue building walls of protection with practical steps.

CHAPTER 7

SUPPLEMENTS, HERBS, AND PEPTIDES TO BOOST THE IMMUNE SYSTEM

I MAGINE LIVING IN a country with virtually no military presence on its borders. No checkpoints, no walls, no fences, no protection. That nation would be wide open to attack and infiltration. Yet in some ways that's how the American population lives, nutritionally speaking. We feel and look OK because we're getting plenty of calories, and our bodies make do with the nutrients we give them. But in truth our immune defenses are down. We are nutritionally deficient. Our bodies are open to pandemic attack.

Earlier I compared our diets to the supply lines that a military force requires to fight and win battles. Supplements are a strategic part of these supply lines. For most people a good diet is not enough to raise the shields of protection in their immune systems. Rather, we need to equip our bodies with the specific vitamins, minerals, and more to strengthen key immune responses. I compare it to a military crisis where all branches of the military are called into active duty, along with the National Guard, Coast Guard, Homeland Security, local police forces, sheriffs, firefighters, and more. When a pandemic hits, we need every advantage we can get—and not only during a pandemic. Preparation and mobilization begin before infectious outbreaks ever take place. Nutritional health should be a lifestyle.

A deficiency of virtually any single nutrient can significantly impair immunity, and so I urge you to take these vitamins and minerals, and consider one of the immune-boosting herbs and a peptide I will discuss below. These will supercharge your immune system, not just in preparation for pandemics, but for optimum health and enjoyment of everyday life.[1]

I also encourage everyone to take a good-quality multivitamin that provides the recommended daily intake of vitamin A, the B vitamins, vitamin E, magnesium, copper, iodine, and omega 3 fats. Even though these didn't make the top list of supplements, they are honorable mentions and important to optimize immune function.

Let's start with what I call the silver bullet for immune function.

THYMOSIN ALPHA 1

I consider thymosin alpha 1 more important than any nutrient for the immune system. Nothing else boosts immune function like it. "Thymosin alpha 1...is a peptide, or small protein, produced naturally by the thymus gland."[2] As I said earlier, the thymus is where T cells are trained and sent into action.

We produce a significant amount of thymosin alpha 1 as children, but as we age we produce less and less. Most people have deficient amounts of thymosin alpha 1 after age sixty, and the immune system effectiveness decreases, and we get more infections and more cancers as we age.[3] This is why people over sixty often need a high-dose flu vaccine with much more of that antigen to elicit an immune response. The thymus has atrophied.

Thymosin alpha 1 stimulates the production of white blood cells that kill viruses in the human body.[4]

Taking it helps to boost the function of the thymus. It's simply amazing. I call it the super-immune booster. It has no side effects and may be the most innocuous prescribed medicine I know of. When you get on thymosin alpha 1, your thymus becomes like a teenager's thymus. Anyone over sixty years of age should seriously consider taking it, and yet so few people have heard of it.

Low amounts of thymosin alpha 1 also leave us more vulnerable to the "cytokine storm" reaction, which works against our recovery from infection. In case you didn't know it, cytokines are defined as "a group of proteins made by the immune system that act as chemical messengers."[5] A cytokine storm is what happens when your immune system goes into high gear and damages your lungs or other organs. It is your immune system overreacting and producing excessive inflammation, usually in the lungs. A cytokine storm is defined as "a severe immune reaction in which the body releases too many cytokines into the blood too quickly."[6] This is what caused some people to be put on ventilators during COVID-19.

The book *The Great Influenza* describes it vividly:

> Dr. Roy Grist, one of the army physicians at the hospital, wrote a colleague, "These men start with what appears to be an ordinary attack of LaGrippe or Influenza, and when brought to the Hosp. they very rapidly develop the most vicious type of Pneumonia that has ever been seen. Two hours after admission they have the Mahogany spots over the cheek bones, and a few hours later you can begin to see the Cyanosis extending from their ears and spreading all over the face, until it is hard to distinguish the coloured men from the white."[7]

The lungs become the battleground and victims of both the virus and the immune system's response. This was evident when examining those who had died from the Spanish flu:

> Normally when the lungs are removed they collapse like deflated balloons. Not now. Now they were full, but not of air.... The bulk of the volume of the lung, was filled with the debris of destroyed cells and with every element of the immune system, from enzymes to white blood cells. And it was filled with blood.[8]

> In the autopsy room they saw the most chilling sights yet. On the table lay the corpse of a young man, not much more than a boy. When he was moved in the slightest degree fluid poured out of his nostrils.[9]

The immune system is designed to function in balance and have a proper reaction without underreacting or overreacting. Thymosin alpha 1 regulates that so that cytokine production is held in check.

"One of the mechanisms in which the COVID-19 virus causes problems in the lung is by inducing what is called 'cytokine storm,'" writes Dr. Teresa Richter, ND. "Cytokines are small proteins that are released from the immune system among other tissues, that send signals to the body to mount a response against infection and to trigger inflammation. This is part of healing. Sometimes the body's response can go into overdrive releasing excessive amounts of cytokines which cause hyper-inflammation that can be seriously harmful. In the case of COVID-19 once the virus enters the lungs, it triggers that cytokine release, which in some people has been excessive leading to more serious illness."[10]

Many doctors don't know about or prescribe thymosin alpha 1, yet it is a key peptide that I recommend to many of my patients sixty years of age or older who want to boost their immune systems. It will need to be prescribed by a physician. I personally administer it to myself two or three times a week, and I usually prescribe thymosin alpha 1 peptide inject 0.5ml SQ two or three times per week.

VITAMIN D$_3$

At the top of my list of recommended supplements is vitamin D$_3$. It has many different functions in the body, and among them is its strong immune-boosting function. Research indicates that T cells must have vitamin D or they will not perform their immune function. "If the T cells cannot find enough vitamin D in the blood, they won't even begin to mobilize."[11] Talk about a necessary vitamin!

One study involving over eleven thousand participants between the ages of zero and ninety-five years found that daily or weekly doses of vitamin D reduced the risk of respiratory tract infections.[12]

About 90 percent of my patients initially have a vitamin D deficiency. Many people think they are getting enough of this key nutrient by drinking fortified milk and spending a few minutes in the sun. But milk does not contain all the vitamin D we need, and most of us don't spend enough time in the sun to produce necessary amounts of vitamin D. Also, sunlight can trigger skin cancer, and in the winter it is difficult for many people to get enough sun to boost vitamin D production. That is probably why vitamin D deficiency and the flu season occur at the same time of year.

Dr. Fuhrman points to a 2006 journal article that stated children who were given interventional vitamin D in the wintertime had fewer viral respiratory infections. Other studies support these results and show people with vitamin D deficiency have an increased risk for acute respiratory illness. Low vitamin D levels have also been associated with an increased risk for influenza.[13]

Another study reviewed vitamin D levels in nearly two hundred healthy adults and showed that those with optimal vitamin D levels reduced their risk of developing acute respiratory tract infections by 50 percent, and they experienced a considerable reduction in the number of days they were ill.[14]

This true story makes the point well:

> Dr. John Cannell was a psychiatrist at the Atascadero State Hospital in California. In 2005, he was in charge of a maximum security facility for the criminally insane.

Knowing that the patients got very little sun exposure, he prescribed high doses of vitamin D to all 32 of his patients. As the winter came the hospital broke-out with a terrible flu epidemic. Dr. Cannell noted that wards all around his got hit hard with the severe flu outbreak but none of his 32 patients caught the flu—even after they mingled with infected inmates from other wards.[15]

I believe that widespread supplementation of vitamin D could prove more effective and affordable than conventional flu vaccines.[16]

Preliminary results from a study by scientists from the Queen Elizabeth Hospital Foundation Trust and the University of East Anglia have linked low levels of vitamin D3 with COVID-19 mortality rates across Europe.

The researchers cataloged the average levels of vitamin D among the citizens of twenty European countries and compared the figures with the relative numbers of COVID-19 deaths in each country.

A statistical test showed a convincing correlation between the figures as populations with below the average concentrations of vitamin D had more deaths from COVID-19. The most vulnerable group of population for COVID-19 was also the one that had the most deficit in vitamin D.[17]

Many health experts recommend daily dosages of 2,000 to 5,000 international units. I boost mine to the high end of their recommendations and take 5,000 international units a day. I recommend supplementing your diet with 2,000 to 5,000 international units of vitamin D per day, or better yet, have your vitamin D_3 level (25OHD3 level) checked by your physician. Optimally the level should be 50–80 ng/mL.

Your immune system will thank you.

ZINC

The other big immune-boosting supplement is zinc. According to a report from Ohio State University, "Zinc deficiency affects about 2 billion people worldwide, including an estimated 40 percent of the elderly in the United States—who are also among the most likely Americans to end up in an ICU."[18]

According to research published in the journal *Cell Reports*, zinc is the key player in keeping our immune response from spiraling out of control and causing excessive inflammation. Scientists say these findings might "help explain why taking zinc tablets at the start of a common cold appears to help stem the effects of the illness."[19]

Indeed, "Among people taking zinc within twenty-four hours of the start of symptoms, the risk of still having symptoms at the seven-day mark was about half that of those not taking zinc," Dr. Fuhrman writes. "[One] review found that not only did zinc reduce the duration and severity of common cold symptoms, but regular zinc use also worked to prevent colds, leading to fewer school absences and less antibiotic use in children. In preventing colds, zinc supplements taken for at least five months reduce the risk of catching a cold to only two-thirds that of people not taking the supplements."[20]

As people age, they are less likely to have adequate zinc levels. That's when they need it most and are most prone to catching a virus. "There is considerable evidence to suggest that regular supplementation with zinc or deliberate consumption of foods rich in zinc is useful to improve immune function and fight off both infections and cancer," writes Dr. Fuhrman. "Studies have been consistently positive in demonstrating that zinc deficiency is associated with an increased incidence and severity of infections and that zinc supplementation is beneficial....Zinc supplementation decreases incidence of pneumonia and antibiotic use....Zinc supplementation decreases the duration of cold and flu by a day or more."[21]

Foods rich in zinc include oysters; Alaskan king crab; beef; raw, unhulled sesame seeds; and raw or roasted pumpkin seeds. "Red meat and poultry provide the majority of zinc in the American diet, according to the National Institutes of Health."[22]

I recommend taking a supplement of 15 mg of zinc per day all year, increasing that to 30 mg with the onset of cold or flu symptoms. Zinc and vitamin D will give attacking infections a powerful one-two punch.

GLUTATHIONE

Glutathione is a powerful antioxidant that is produced in the liver and works throughout the body in cells, tissues, and fluids to detoxify free radicals created from oxygen. "Glutathione has been called the 'mother' of all antioxidants" because it binds and "sticks" to toxins and free radicals of all kinds so that your body can dispose of them. But glutathione also supports the immune system. "When intracellular glutathione level dips, white blood cells called lymphocytes are impaired and viral infections can percolate....Rapid decreases in glutathione levels have been seen after infection with viruses."[23]

According to Dr. Tasreen Alibhai, ND, "Taking Glutathione as a supplement will help to reduce this oxidative stress in your body and particularly on your immune system. The result is a stronger immune system that can help to fight off infections such as the flu virus....Studies have shown Glutathione strengthens T Cell activity in the immune system, which coordinates the attack against viruses and bacteria."[24]

In one study of 262 elderly subjects, glutathione supplementation helped participants to develop far fewer symptoms of the flu and recover much faster.[25]

Another study found that "oxidative stress or other conditions that deplete GSH [glutathione] in the epithelium of the oral, nasal, and upper airway may, therefore, enhance susceptibility to influenza infection."[26]

In a monthlong study by researcher at Penn State, liposomal glutathione helped to elevate the effectiveness of natural killer cells by up to 400 percent.[27]

Glutathione is also able to decrease inflammation in the body. Excessive cytokine release causes the cytokine storm that may lead to pneumonia and is simply excessive inflammation, usually in the lungs. Glutathione helps to quench this inflammation.

How do we get this amazing substance? Foods like broccoli, brussels sprouts, cauliflower, cabbage, and raw garlic, and spices like cinnamon, turmeric, and cardamom stimulate production of glutathione.[28]

Vitamin C and N-acetyl-cysteine (NAC) increase the rate of synthesis of glutathione. I recommend between 500 and 1,000 mg of NAC a day. Cellgevity is my favorite glutathione-boosting supplement, which boosts glutathione 267–292 percent. (See appendix B.)

SELENIUM

Selenium deficiency has a significant impact on the influenza-induced defense responses in human airway epithelial cells, according to one study.[29]

Dietary selenium "strongly influences inflammation and immune responses," according to an article published in *Molecular Nutrition & Food Research*. It boosts the immune system, especially in the elderly, and protects against certain pathogens. "Studies have demonstrated an enhancement of both cell-mediated and humoral immune responses by increasing levels of [selenium] intake."[30]

Selenium deficiency also has been shown to increase susceptibility to viruses such as HIV, and selenium benefits aging immune systems.[31]

Proper levels of selenium and other antioxidants is "especially important for maintaining proper immune responses in aging individuals."[32]

Experts suggest that "good dietary sources of selenium include Brazil nuts, organ meats, muscle meats, poultry, fish, oysters, rolled oats and wheat flour."[33] However, I do not recommend eating organ meats and wheat.

The recommended daily value for selenium is 55 micrograms a day for adults. I place many of my patients on 100 micrograms a day during flu season.

PROBIOTICS

Probiotics are living organisms that improve the health of your gut, specifically the good bacteria in your gut biome. They reduce inflammation, balance your gut bacteria, help train your immune system, strengthen your gut lining, reduce your gut permeability, and help your body digest protein, absorb nutrients better, and fight infection.[34]

Probiotics improve your immune system and strengthen your intestinal wall while they stop, kill, or limit the growth of bad bacteria. Those are great benefits!

I usually put my patients on at least one to two probiotic capsules a day and sometimes more. Sometimes I will use two to four different types of probiotics, depending on the severity of their gut condition. (See appendix B.)

ELDERBERRY

Black elderberry juice is widely used to treat colds and the flu. Studies suggest that black elderberry extract (2 to 3 tablespoons daily for adults and 1 to 4 teaspoons for children, depending on age) can inhibit the growth of influenza viruses, shorten the duration of symptoms, and enhance antibody levels against the virus.[35]

The purple pigments in elderberry seem to be responsible for helping fight the flu. "These pigments, known as anthocyanins, are powerfully antioxidant, but also appear to possess anti-viral activity."[36]

Dr. Fuhrman writes that "elderberry has been demonstrated to inhibit the adhesion of the virus to the cell receptors. When the virus is inhibited from entering cells, it cannot replicate itself, and this can lessen the seriousness of the infection."[37]

In *Prevention* magazine, Chris Kilham writes that "elderberry is widely available as a liquid, capsule, and tablet. The most tested elderberry preparation for fighting flu is called Sambucol.... It is most effective when taken at the first sign of flu."[38]

Don't eat elderberries raw, because they can cause vomiting. Rather, take them in syrup or pill form, like Sambucol. I take it even before I feel something coming on. Elderberry syrups tend to have too much sugar, so I don't favor them. I take it in pill form.

But make this natural supplement part of your immune defense supply system. (See appendix B.) The dose of elderberry in capsule form is usually 150–175 mg two times a day.

VITAMIN C

I have used IV vitamin C in high doses for decades to treat viral diseases. Many animal studies show that vitamin C plays a role in preventing, shortening, and alleviating diverse infections, and controlled studies in humans have shown that vitamin C shortens and alleviates the common cold. Five controlled trials found significant effects of vitamin C against pneumonia.[39]

> "Our bodies don't make vitamin C, but we need it for immune function," according to Harvard Health.[40]

Vitamin C kills microbes and helps produce B and T cells. People with vitamin C deficiency, one study found, "tend to have impaired immunity and are more susceptible to infection, and supplementing with vitamin C can help prevent respiratory infections—like the flu."[41]

A number of studies on vitamin C show that "therapeutic doses (3–4 grams a day) of the vitamin taken at the onset of a cold could reduce its duration, and reduce fever, chills and chest pain. Vitamin C can…support white blood cells' migration to the site of infections and their ability to generate free radicals that can kill microbes.…When healthy volunteers supplemented with vitamin C, their neutrophils—a white blood cell—had enhanced activity."[42]

According to Harvard Health, "taking at least 200 mg of vitamin C per day did appear to reduce the duration of cold symptoms by an average of 8% in adults and 14% in children.…If you want the benefits of vitamin C, you'll need to consume it every day, and not just at the start of cold symptoms."[43]

Vitamin C is found in citrus fruits, strawberries, green vegetables, and tomatoes. "Liposomal vitamin C is an advanced form of vitamin C designed for better absorption and utilization within the body. Liposomes are small spherical cells that are composed of an outer layer of oils derived from either sunflower or soy." The water-soluble vitamin C is protected within this compartment. "The bioavailability of liposomal vitamin C is significantly greater than regular vitamin C [and] is taken up into the body at almost double the level that of regular vitamin C."[44]

ASTRAGALUS ROOT

Astragalus root is an herb that boosts cell-mediated immunity and appears to raise white blood cell counts. It has long been used in traditional Chinese medicine to treat viruses. "Clinical studies in China have validated it is effective when used as a preventive measure against the common cold. It has also been shown to reduce the duration and severity of symptoms in acute treatment of the common cold.... It appears to stimulate white blood cells to engulf and destroy invading organisms."[45]

According to an article published by Penn State Hershey Medical Center, "In the United States, researchers have looked at astragalus as a possible treatment for people whose immune systems have been weakened by chemotherapy or radiation. In these studies, astragalus supplements seem to help people recover faster and live longer." Several studies show that astragalus acts like an antioxidant and may help treat heart disease. According to other studies, it may help lower cholesterol levels.[46]

I recommend taking 250–500 mg of astragalus, three to four times a day, if this is an herb you choose to take. I don't recommend taking all three herbs listed here—astragalus, Andrographis paniculata, and cat's claw—but rather just one of them. Take caution if you have an autoimmune disease. Some immune-boosting herbs can worsen autoimmune diseases.

ANDROGRAPHIS PANICULATA

Andrographolide, a substance derived from plants, is known for its anti-inflammatory effects and seems to enhance cytotoxic T cells and natural killer (NK) cells.[47]

One study concluded that "andrographolide treatment could increase the survival rate, diminish lung pathology, decrease the virus loads and the inflammatory cytokines expression induced by infection," and in combination with other treatments "might be a promising therapeutic approach for influenza."[48]

Another article reports that "in India, andrographis was widely credited for arresting the 1919 Indian flu epidemic, says J. Hancke, M.D., with the Max Planck Institute, who led two double-blind placebo-controlled studies on the herb in Sweden....In one study involving 107 18-year-old students, half took 200 mg of andrographis (standardized to contain 5.6 percent andrographolides—the active constituent) daily for three months. The other half took placebo. By the end of the trial, 16 students in the andrographis group had developed colds, compared with 33 students in the control group. In another study, andrographis reduced cold symptom severity....Of 158 adults with colds, participants given 1,200 mg daily of andrographis (standardized to contain 5.6 percent andrographolides) experienced significant improvements by the second day of treatment, and improved further by day four, compared with participants who received placebo. The symptoms that improved the most were earache, sleeplessness, nasal drainage and sore throat, though other cold symptoms improved as well."[49]

I recommend taking 500 mg of andrographis two or three times a day in capsule form, if you elect to. (See appendix B.)

CAT'S CLAW

This popular herb from the Amazon rain forest is widely considered to be a powerful immunity enhancer and has been used to treat many ailments for hundreds of years. Many people take it to reduce the risk of getting sick and to reduce the severity of illness.[50] According to research, "Cat's claw offers powerful immune support and boosts activity of immune cells such as B- and T-lymphocytes. It stimulates the ability of white blood cells to gobble up invaders…and enhances cytokines that enhance immune function. It has been shown to strongly stimulate immune cells called macrophages. In a study of adult males, those who supplemented with cat's claw for six months saw a boost in their white blood cell count." It also functions as an anti-inflammatory.[51]

I recommend taking 250–500 mg of cat's claw twice per day.

OLEANDRIN

In addition to the supplements already in this chapter, this late-breaking new supplement is so important I decided to include it as a bonus.

An extremely important antiviral supplement, and perhaps the best of all, is oleandrin, from the oleander plant, which is a native American plant. Oleandrin is also a cardiac glycoside, which is used therapeutically to treat irregular heart rhythms and congestive heart failure.

Oleandrin has demonstrated strong antiviral activity against numerous enveloped viruses, including COVID-19, HIV-1, CMV, Ebola, Marburg, alphavirus (which causes encephalitis), and human T-Cell leukemia virus type 1. Oleandrin also passes through the blood-brain barrier and enters the brain. An enveloped virus means that the outer layer of the virus is a lipid (fatty) membrane, which is taken from the host cell. Oleandrin prevents viruses from forming their protective envelope, resulting in viral progeny (viral shedding) with a significantly impaired ability to infect. The envelope protein is essential for a virus to bind to target cells and infect them.[52]

In vitro studies of oleandrin by the University of Texas Medical Branch (UTMB) showed a dramatic reduction in infectious virus production using nontoxic concentrations of oleandrin. UTMB is performing more studies to determine how long after infection with COVID-19 oleandrin can be applied to cells and still suppress viral replication and rescue cells from COVID-19-induced death. Preliminary results look very promising. You will soon be able to purchase oleandrin online under the name Serrativir, produced by Phoenix Biotechnology.

LESS SUGAR, PLEASE

Consuming high amounts of sugar weakens the immune response and creates a favorable environment for a flu virus to take hold. Several trials have shown that the ability of some white blood cells to ingest and engulf bacteria, fungi, and other pathogens dropped by almost 50 percent after consumption of 100-gram doses of simple sugars, such as sucrose, glucose, fructose, orange juice, and honey. The immunosuppressive effects of the sugar lasted several hours.[53]

One way to help your body be a "no-go" zone for viruses and other invaders is by consuming only very small amounts of sugar—especially when outbreaks and infections are threatening.

By marshaling your troops and supplying them well with a good diet and immune-boosting supplements, you create effective borders and barriers in the form of a strong and capable immune system response.

Now let's look at the social and interactive aspects of pandemic protection—how to engage with others safely in public, how to shop for groceries, and much more.

CHAPTER 8

AN OUNCE OF PREVENTION IS WORTH A POUND OF CURE (SOCIAL DISTANCING)

FOR MANY PEOPLE, the idea of "social distancing," wearing masks and gloves in public, and staying home for weeks on end due to the coronavirus was new and somewhat strange. Some people resisted these ideas. Some embraced new health practices right away. As a country, and a world, we began to figure out what a coordinated, community-level response to a virulent pandemic looks like.

While many people adopted healthy procedures and lifestyles right away, others learned the hard way, though out of ignorance and not malice. One church in Arkansas's Cleburne County didn't want to cancel its services in early March 2020, when the coronavirus didn't seem to many people to be a threat. The church went ahead and hosted a special children's ministry event. According to the Family Research Council, "The result was catastrophic."[1]

Dozens of people linked to the church came down with the coronavirus—including Pastor Mark Palenske and his wife. He posted on Facebook that "the intensity of this virus has been underestimated by so many, and I continue to ask that each of you take it very seriously. An act of wisdom and restraint on your part can be the blessing that preserves the health of someone else."[2] The situation in Cleburne County became so serious "that judges and other officials had to close their offices completely."[3]

In Italy, a larger gathering had much the same effect. The Associated Press called the February 19, 2020, soccer game in San Siro Stadium the biggest in Atalanta's history. It pitted the local team against a Spanish team from Valencia. More than forty thousand fans jammed the stadium, but the match became a "biological bomb" according to one respiratory specialist. Experts say it was the primary reason that the nearby city of Bergamo became an epicenter of the virus, and more than a third of the Spanish soccer team later tested positive for COVID-19. Headlines called it "Game Zero."[4]

These kinds of events showed all of us a world few had lived in before—a world where even going into public might cause us to become infected by a powerful new virus. Dr. Nikita Desai, a pulmonologist at Cleveland Clinic, told NBC News, "Remember that transmission is not just person to person, it's also place to place. Everywhere you go, you might leave virus and then someone else may come and pick it up."[5]

In the Western world the virus often spread by way of mass gatherings—on cruise ships, at choir rehearsals, at ski resorts, even in a prison. "'It's very much driven by the context of a gathering' and how people disperse after it's over, spreading it to other individuals or groups," said Dr. Michael Ryan, executive director of the WHO Health Emergencies Programme, at a press conference on Feb. 24," 2020, according to NPR.[6]

One group of vacationers was staying in a ski chalet in a French resort near Mont Blanc when another visitor arrived, a British man who had attended a business conference in Singapore. Soon after this, new cases began to pop up in the UK and France, linked to the interactions at the ski resort.[7]

A similar thing happened in an Austrian ski town where an outbreak occurred. The country of Norway concluded that nearly 40 percent of its more than 1,400 infections at the time originated in Austria, many of them in the ski town where travelers from

Iceland infected with coronavirus arrived and inadvertently spread the illness.[8]

At Rikers Island Jail in New York the victims had little choice. Within a twelve-day period cases among prisoners at Rikers approached two hundred, according to Ross MacDonald, the jail's chief physician—and the infection rate for New York City's jails was nearly 4 percent.[9]

In a rather sad story, a man who had been exposed to the coronavirus and was feeling sick "hid his symptoms from the staff at a New York hospital so he could join his expectant wife in the maternity center. He confessed only when his wife began to show symptoms of COVID-19 shortly after giving birth at Strong Memorial Hospital."[10]

As strong as our immune systems are through healthy eating, good sleep, exercise, peaceful thinking, and supplements, none of us should walk around believing we are totally invincible. Nobody is a superhero. The Bible strongly encourages prudence, which is the deliberate avoidance of danger and trouble. While I believe I am much more likely to pass along a virus than to feel its effects— and I believe the same is true for anyone practicing the lifestyle outlined in this book—part of protecting ourselves from pandemics is to not be reckless or proud. We can feel very confident in our ability to combat infections while also taking safeguards that only serve to make us safer.

It's also a way of serving others during a crisis. Think of the people in your life who are older or whose immune systems are compromised somehow. Think even of the strangers you might come into brief contact with in public whose lives could be radically changed if they were to become infected by a powerful invader you passed on to them. For these reasons I strongly encourage all of us to practice preventative measures in public places and at home through such things as social distancing, handwashing, and use of sanitizer, gloves, and glasses or goggles, among other things. Consider it another line of defense so that our bodies can win the war without even fighting.

As an example, let me show you what a normal shopping outing looks like for me in the midst of a pandemic.

DR. C AT THE STORE

I keep in my car a roll of paper towels, surgical gloves, hand sanitizer, goggles, and a face mask. On the way to the store I listen to uplifting Christian music or talk radio. My heart is at ease and confident of the Lord's protection in all circumstances as I head out to do a little shopping.

When I park at the store and turn the car off, I take off my sunglasses and put on the nice-fitting protective glasses I bought at Home Depot. They fit beautifully, are comfortable, and even look stylish, like a pair of fitness glasses. The most important thing is that they seal my eyes and are comfortable. At one point I had a pair of goggles that were so uncomfortable that I sometimes didn't wear them. My present pair feels good and seals my eyes beautifully.

Next I put my surgery mask on. I use about one mask per day and keep it lying upside down on the dashboard so UV light from the sun can kill germs. It's best not to touch the mask itself, so I'm careful how I take it off and put it on. I touch the ear loops, not the mask, and slip them over my ears.

Then I put my gloves on and put a little bottle of hand sanitizer in my pocket. I have plenty of hand sanitizer because I buy it in big containers, which I use to fill up smaller ones that are easier to carry. I have these small containers available for my staff and my family as well.

Whenever I put on surgical gloves, I'm reminded of a

powerful story related in the book *None of These Diseases* by S. I. McMillen. In 1847, in the Vienna General Hospital in Austria, an obstetrician-gynecologist named Ignaz Semmelweis was troubled by the number of pregnant women dying of "labor fever." Germs were unknown at the time. Illness was blamed on bad air or atmospheric conditions. Medical students regularly conducted autopsies of dead women with bare hands, coming into contact with pus, then rinsed the blood from their hands, wiped their hands with a rag, and went immediately to the maternity ward to deliver babies and conduct internal exams of pregnant women.[11] It's hard for us to imagine this happening, but it was standard scientific practice at the time.

Semmelweis made the correlation between unwashed hands and the transmission of illness—a controversial idea in that day. He noticed that women who had more internal exams were more likely to die of labor fever. So were women whose babies were delivered by a doctor rather than a midwife. The difference, he observed, was that doctors conducted autopsies and midwives did not. Semmelweis began insisting that his students wash their hands in chlorinated water between autopsies and exams. As a result, mortality rates among pregnant women in his hospital dropped from 18 percent to 1 percent. Semmelweis had similar results in other hospitals where his handwashing practices were instituted. After facing open rejection of his theories for years, the medical establishment finally embraced the practice of handwashing and antisepsis, and of course, many fewer diseases were passed among patients, doctors, and nurses.[12]

Wearing gloves works by the same principle.

As I get out of my car wearing glasses, a mask, and gloves, I take a couple of paper towels with me in case I have to open a door. I may use one to wipe down the shopping cart too. Once inside the store, I keep my distance from everyone and don't dillydally. My goal is not to go up and down aisles seeing what's on sale or what's new. During a pandemic I want to get what I need and get out. I'm usually in the store for around five to ten minutes total.

Common recommendations during COVID-19 said to keep a distance of six feet from others, but the virus was shown to linger in the air for hours. I read a study that particles from a sneeze can travel twenty-seven feet![13] Those particles can stay airborne for hours and get in your eyes, nose, or mouth. You may be walking through a store and think you're totally safe but you're walking in a hot zone.

As Dr. Fuhrman writes, "Viruses are primarily spread via hand-to-face contact. They can also be spread when a sick person coughs or sneezes, aerosolizing the virus so others inhale it. A person can be contagious the day before he or she develops symptoms and for seven to ten days after symptoms first develop."[14]

One sobering real-life occurrence during COVID-19 drives the point home. In Washington state in early March, a choral group decided to hold its weekly rehearsal though the virus was already causing some concern. The county hadn't reported any cases, and schools and businesses remained open. Sixty singers met at Mount Vernon Presbyterian Church, were offered hand sanitizer at the door, and refrained from the usual hugs and handshakes. The singers tried to maintain a certain distance from each other during their two-and-a-half-hour practice.

Three weeks later, forty-five of the sixty were diagnosed with COVID-19 or had symptoms, three were hospitalized, and two were dead. County health officials concluded that the virus was transmitted through the air from people without symptoms. Participants said no one at the rehearsal was coughing or sneezing or appeared ill. According to the *Los Angeles Times*, "Experts said the choir outbreak is consistent with a growing body of evidence that the virus can be transmitted through aerosols—particles smaller than 5 micrometers that can float in the air for minutes or longer."[15]

That's a great example of what I mean about the virus traveling through the air and staying there longer than we might expect. Although I keep my distance from people and move quickly to do my shopping, I never become tense, angry, or anxious. Though I'm wearing a mask and people can't see me smiling, I still am polite, courteous, and exude the peace of God. During the COVID-19 crisis, I had never seen such fear on the faces of people in line. They were jittery, fidgety, curt, inwardly focused emotionally, worried about getting the products they needed, and sometimes just plain selfish. Others, of course, were generous and friendly. It was like two worlds colliding. When I'm in public during a pandemic, I remain calm and at peace. I believe we can powerfully change atmospheres and strengthen others with the love, joy, and peace we carry with us, as we looked at in chapter 5.

When I am finished shopping, I stand in line a good distance from the person in front of me. When it's my turn, I put my items on the conveyor belt and use the plastic divider. I'm not afraid to touch these things, because I have gloves on. The bagger bags my groceries. I pay with a credit card, take the paper bags they give me, thank them, and walk through the automatic door to my car. Once there, I put the groceries in the back seat, then pull out my hand sanitizer and wipe down the credit card and set it to the side to let it dry. The clerk who may have handled the credit card has handled thousands of others. They don't really have the option to sanitize their hands between every transaction.

Some people get lax when they get back to their cars. They take their masks and goggles off, rub their eyes, noses, or mouths, and introduce the virus back into their systems after leaving the war zone. But this is no time to let your guard down. Back when SARS was breaking out, many of the victims were healthcare workers. Apparently they became infected when they were careless or took shortcuts when removing their protective equipment. We don't want to lose the battle at the last moment.

I remove my gloves and throw them away. I then take the glasses off and put them in the passenger seat or middle console. I carefully remove my mask, handling only the ear loops, and put it on the dashboard upside down. I sometimes spray the inside of my mask with hydrogen peroxide and let it dry in the sunlight. I remind myself not to touch my face inadvertently. I then apply hand sanitizer to my hands, making sure I get between my fingers and under my fingernails. I keep my fingernails very short because viruses can hide under the nails.

If I have to fill up with gas on the way home, I take a sheet of paper towels and grab the gas handle with them. I believe that gas handles almost certainly carry whatever pandemic is spreading. At least I treat them as if they do. I recently heard of a healthy football player who believes he contracted COVID-19 from a gas handle; he spent five days in the hospital.[16]

As soon as I get home, I take my shoes off and leave them at the door because the virus could be on the bottom of my shoes. I put the grocery bags not on the kitchen counter but in an area where we keep our personal items. The reason is that I want to make sure nothing on the boxes touches our kitchen counters. During outbreaks Mary and I are extra diligent about making our kitchen an infection-free zone. We wipe the counters down with Clorox spray a few times a day. We don't allow purses, cell phones, grocery bags, computers, or anything like that in the kitchen because viruses can survive for days on these items, and it's easy to carry it from one place to another without realizing it. We don't always live with this degree of vigilance, but rules change during pandemics.

Before unbagging the groceries, I wash my hands thoroughly with foam soap. According to the Mayo Clinic, "over-the-counter antibacterial soaps are no more effective at killing germs than is regular soap." They recommend following these steps:

- "Wet your hands with clean, running water—either warm or cold.
- Apply soap and lather well.
- Rub your hands vigorously for at least twenty seconds. Remember to scrub all surfaces, including the backs of your hands, wrists, between your fingers, and under your fingernails.
- Rinse well.
- Dry your hands with a clean towel or air-dry them."[17]

Some are curious about how handwashing works. It's all in the oils. Most of the unwanted stuff that sticks to our hands, whether it's a virus or just plain dirt, does so due to the oils on our skin. Soap or hand sanitizer attaches to oil particles or breaks down the oil so that the germs and dirt wash away.[18]

Soap works well not just for removing viruses but for killing them. One helpful newspaper report described it well: "The virus is a self-assembled nanoparticle in which the weakest link is the lipid (fatty) bilayer. Soap dissolves the fat membrane and the virus falls apart like a house of cards and dies—or rather, we should say it becomes inactive, as viruses aren't really alive.... The soap not only loosens the 'glue' between the virus and the skin but also the Velcro-like interactions that hold the proteins, lipids and RNA in the virus together. Alcohol-based products, which pretty much includes all 'disinfectant' products, contain a high-percentage alcohol solution (typically 60–80% ethanol) and kill viruses in a similar fashion. But soap is better because you only need a fairly small amount of soapy water, which, with rubbing, covers your entire hand easily."[19]

I don't recommend using only water, but if there is no soap available for some reason, just rubbing your hands together under the water is helpful. "A 2011 study from researchers at the London School of Tropical Hygiene found that washing with water alone reduced bacteria on hands to about one-quarter of their prewash state. Washing with soap and water brought bacterial counts down to about 8% of where they were before washing."[20]

Make sure to dry your hands vigorously with a paper towel, an action that removes even more germs.[21]

After washing and drying my hands, I put the groceries away—eggs in the fridge, frozen goods in the freezer, and so on. I'm not worried about catching a virus from food containers because it has never been shown to be transmitted this way. It is potentially possible but very improbable. I also wipe off the doorknob on my back door, which is the one we use the most, and any other outdoor doorknobs, if used. I do this with disinfectant wipes one or two times per day or as needed. I also wipe off my car door handle as needed.

I throw away the shopping bags, then go to the living room to relax! That is what my shopping routine looks like during a pandemic. The point is to take simple, practical steps to raise a physical barrier between you and the virus or contagion, but not to feel strange or anxious about what you are doing.

Remember that peace of mind is huge in keeping our immune systems performing well.

PANDEMIC PRACTICES

There are other things we can do as well because there is no silver bullet for defeating pandemics. It's an all-of-the-above approach. I sometimes see people taking great care to wear masks and sanitize their shopping carts, but then they buy nonnutritious food, and by all appearances they aren't getting much exercise. Hand sanitizer alone can't fix that.

During pandemics the right thing to do is to practice public prevention. Exercise restraint and wisdom until the crisis passes. Take walks and smile and wave to others, but keep your distance for the time being. Always cover your cough or sneeze with a tissue and then throw it in the trash, or cough or sneeze in the bend of your elbow. Avoid touching your eyes, nose, and mouth with unwashed hands. Have plenty of hand sanitizer, alcohol, gloves, masks or scarves, and safety goggles on hand.

During the Spanish flu of 1918–20, the US Surgeon General offered this advice to avoid the deadly influenza. Some of it remains relevant today, and some is a product of its time. He wrote:

> Avoid needless crowding....Smother your coughs and sneezes....Your nose not your mouth was made to breathe thru....Remember the 3 Cs, clean mouth, clean skin, and clean clothes....Food will win the war....[H]elp by choosing and chewing your food well....Wash your hands before eating....Don't let the waste products of digestion accumulate....Avoid tight clothes, tight shoes, tight gloves—seek to make nature your ally not your prisoner....When the air is pure breathe all of it you can—breathe deeply.[22]

At our house, we stopped having guests over during COVID-19. Rather, we connected with more people online, and that was a real blessing. We may have socialized more than we did before the pandemic!

We continued to have our kids and grandkids over. They had to abide by the house rules and take their shoes off at the front door, and wash their hands, especially before eating. We made it enjoyable by humming the song "Happy Birthday to You."

If you find yourself needing a face mask and don't have the option to go out and buy one, it's easy to make one with homemade materials. I saw an online video where someone used two strong paper towels, folded accordion-style as if you were making a fan. Staple a separate rubber band to each end of the paper towels and use them for ear loops. Then unbunch the paper towels and wear them over your face. You may need to cut the paper towel to fit your face. It's effective and simple!

Some people feel they need to shower more often during a pandemic, but it's not necessary and could be harmful. You only need to shower daily at most. Some people shower so much that they needlessly remove the good bacteria from their skin. We need our good bacteria to suppress viral growth. Use soap mainly on your private parts and armpits. Think of it as probiotic washing.

Speaking of which, the frequency of the need to wash hands can leave them dry and cracked during a pandemic. To alleviate this side effect, I use straight extra-virgin organic coconut oil as a moisturizer two or three times a day. It's great for your skin and helps keep viruses from getting into dry, cracked areas.

After pandemics pass, there is no reason to keep wearing masks and staying far away from each other in public. We don't need to permanently change lifestyles and practice preventative social distancing. I have one colleague who cleans her hands with sanitizer after touching virtually anything, and as a result her hands are constantly chapped—and she's riddled with anxiety! Our lives are not always defined by avoiding a disease, and we can thank God that all pandemics pass at some point or other. Sometimes the summer heat and humidity knock them out. Sometimes the population builds up an immunity, or an effective vaccine is created.

Until the pandemic eases, be prudent in preventing it from entering your body or your home by taking these commonsense measures.

CHAPTER 9

RESIST FEAR AND FEED YOUR FAITH

URING THE COVID-19 shutdown I still had to travel by airplane for work, and much of what I saw—and felt—amazed me. The nearly empty airports and trams in Atlanta and Dallas were eerie and interesting. What surprised me most was that among those people still traveling during the worst of the pandemic, the fear level was often toxic. Many seemed afraid to interact at all, locked in behind their goggles and masks. It was like a living picture of how people avoided the sick during the Great Plague of London. On one jumbo jet I counted around twenty people total, and as you would imagine, they each took seats far away from each other. We had multiple rows to ourselves, which wasn't bad!

During a pandemic or not, when I travel I have a well-tested strategy to help bring peace to public places—and that strategy came in especially handy then. My method is simple, but I can testify that it works! Here it is: When I travel, I wear a T-shirt that has the entire chapter of Psalm 23 printed in large letters all over it. "The Lord is my shepherd, I shall not want. He maketh me lie down in green pastures....Yea, though I walk through the valley of the shadow of death, I will fear no evil; for thou art with me," and so on. During the COVID-19 pandemic I wore this T-shirt on flights as I usually did, and it amazed me to see people's expressions change as they read the words on my shirt. Their icy fear melted just a bit. Some started quoting it aloud, and when they did, I quoted the next part back to them! Peace settled on them in place of the cloud of uncertainty and dread.

More than one passenger and flight attendant approached me to say, "I'm so encouraged by your shirt." Even TSA people told me, "Man, I love your shirt." Sometimes when I saw them looking, I pointed to different areas on the shirt and said, "Look at this promise here, and this one over here." It created a wide-open door to share the Word of God with them, giving the only sure strength and peace we have in hard times.

FAITH IN ACTION

I shared earlier about replacing stress with peace, and gave ways to cultivate healthy thought patterns that boost your immune system. Here I want to go deeper down to the only true foundation for a positive, immune-boosting outlook during a pandemic: faith in God and His biblical promises. Faith underlies all healthy thinking and living, and I strongly encourage you to base every thought and opinion you have on the written Word of God. Get it inside of your mind and heart and let it define you. When fear presents itself you will find yourself saying, "God has not given me a spirit of fear, but of power, love, and a sound mind." You might surprise yourself with what comes out! I guarantee that your faith will form a powerful shield of protection, spiritually and physically.

Recently I read about twenty-seven-year-old Yvonne Walters of Slidell, Louisiana, who thought she had the flu and went to the emergency room—where doctors almost immediately emergency intubated her and eventually put her into a medically induced coma because she had COVID-19. Yvonne eventually recovered, and during the scariest time of her bout with the infection, Yvonne's mother, Raquelle, "leaned heavily on her faith," according to a news report. "We just kind of went into faith mode prayer mode believe totally in God, no doubt, no wavering," said Raquelle.[1]

After coming out of the coma and beating the virus, Yvonne said, "I feel like there's power in prayer and don't ever doubt that there is a God because I know that my mom she's the strongest woman I know and I had no idea that so many people were praying for me."[2]

In Cleveland, a patient who beat COVID-19 left a handwritten message of faith on the wall of his isolation room for the ICU medical staff at the Cleveland Clinic to read. The message read in part, "Today I leave this ICU a changed person, hopefully for the better, not only because of your medical healing & God's direction and guidance, but with the fact of knowing that there are such wonderful people dedicated to the care and concern of others. God bless each of you."[3]

There were many uplifting stories like that during COVID-19 of people young and old healing from the virus. The words of Dr. Fuhrman represent my firm view that "even the more virulent and dangerous flu strains, such as the avian flu, stand little chance against a truly healthy immune system."[4]

Our immune systems thrive when we stand on the Word of God and declare His truth over any potential threat.

VOICING YOUR FAITH

Our biggest task as believers is to not let a pandemic build a stronghold in our thought lives. Fear acts like enemy propaganda on our health, weakening us, making us afraid, inviting illness and defeat. I recommend that every believer quote specific scriptures aloud throughout the day, multiple times, meditating on them, and ending the day by speaking them aloud again. The Word of God builds a fortress of faith in our minds and lives. It breaks down any strongholds of fear and worry that the enemy may have begun to build through news reports, social media, or your interactions with fear-filled people.

To live by faith is to literally choose life over death. Romans 8:5–6 says, "For those who live according to the flesh set their minds on the things of the flesh, but those who live according to the Spirit, the things of the Spirit. For to be carnally minded is death, but to be spiritually minded is life and peace." Our response to pandemics should not be like the world's response. Even if we have to get up early to go to the store to buy supplies, or cancel travel and business plans, or wear protective gear, we should not be anxious like other people might be. Peace can spread through a group of people just as fast as anxiety can. A pandemic is our time to be leaders, tone-setters, atmosphere-changers, and overcomers in our communities and families.

A great passage to read aloud during a pandemic is one that many were quoting and preaching from during COVID-19: Psalm 91. Read it aloud and insert your name and the names of your loved ones wherever it says "you." For example, verse 3 would read, "Surely He shall deliver me and my family from the snare of the fowler." Let's practice the whole thing together (based on the NLT):

> Those who live in the shelter of the Most High will find rest in the shadow of the Almighty.
>
> This I declare about the LORD: He alone is my refuge, my place of safety; he is my God, and I trust him.
>
> For he will rescue me and my family (name each member) from every trap and protect me and my family (name each member again) from deadly disease.
>
> He will cover me and my family (you know what to do) with his feathers. He will shelter me and my family with his wings. His faithful promises are my armor and protection.
>
> Do not be afraid of the terrors of the night, nor the arrow that flies in the day.
>
> Do not dread the disease that stalks in darkness, nor the disaster that strikes at midday.

Though a thousand fall at my side, though ten thousand are dying around me, these evils will not touch me or my family.

No plague will come near my home!

Do this with other psalms, and you will feel the results in your mind, emotions, and body!

Another foundational verse for immune-boosting faith is 2 Timothy 1:7. Again, personalize it by saying, "God has not given me a spirit of fear, but of power, love, and a sound mind." Another great one is Philippians 4:6–7 (NIV), which you can read aloud this way: "I am not anxious about anything, but in every situation, by prayer and petition, with thanksgiving, I present my requests to God. And the peace of God, which transcends all understanding, will guard my heart and my mind in Christ Jesus."

There are numerous places in God's Word where it says "Fear not." Find those and make them your own. Then find and personalize other promises in the Bible. I call this reframing according to God's Word. It is the God-given way to use your faith to quench fiery darts of doubt, and supercharge your immune system in the process.

Take Ground

I encourage you to go further. Instead of just holding your ground, use times of pandemic to gain ground in your faith. Use any extra time you have to study a specific book or theme of the Bible in greater depth. Take an online Bible course to deepen your knowledge and bolster your faith. Connect with others by holding Zoom Bible studies, or creating prayer groups by conference call or text. This might even be a good time to reconnect with people with whom you have a strained relationship. Maybe forgiveness is needed. Maybe there just needs to be a good, positive conversation to say, "I care for you and hope you're doing well." Take what the enemy intended for ill in the pandemic and use it to advance God's kingdom in your life.

Make sure to keep a journal of these things to encourage yourself and to record the growth that happened during that season. Fill it with statements of gratitude and praise, testimonies of God's faithfulness and protection during the crisis, and anything you feel God speaking to your heart. These will fill your heart with faith, gratitude, and a sense of celebration when you read over them.

All of that will enhance your immune response and contribute to overall physical health.

LOOK FOR MIRACLES

In addition to looking for good-news stories of recovery, pay attention to miracles happening in your own life. For example, during a particularly deep recession some years back, my practice went from fully booked-up to very few patients. I had to reinvent my career and make some changes, which turned out to be much better for my future. I also used my extra time to start a medical clinic for the poor in Sanford, Florida.

During COVID-19 the same thing happened. Early on I asked the Lord how He wanted to use this in my life to move me forward, and the Lord gave me a word: telemedicine. I was very excited, not least because I then had a project to do during the lockdown! Right away I could see that telemedicine is a big part of the future of medicine. While I was limited on the number of patients I could see during the pandemic, since many of my patients fly in from all over the US and the world, I could treat them through a video screen. Neither of us had to wear a mask. The patient didn't have to go into public and be worried about catching something.

Of course, I couldn't check their vital signs, but I was amazed at how much I could diagnose through a screen.

For example, one patient had a horrible rash on her face. It was easy to tell it was rosacea, and I knew how to help her. Suddenly my practice became global, and while a lot of doctors were scrambling to fill the void in their schedules, I was excited to see new opportunities open up right before me. It all began by getting a word from God about the situation, then acting on it by faith.

I believe God has plans for you in every crisis, every pandemic, every difficulty that comes upon the world, to advance you and take you higher in every way. Stand on faith and watch the miracles He performs for you.

CHAPTER 10

PROPHETIC PERSPECTIVE ON PANDEMICS

IN JANUARY 2020 I began to feel a nudge in my spirit to sell our house. It didn't make a lot of sense, but the urgency grew stronger within me.

Our house at that time was out in the country, near a lake and far away from the city of Dallas-Fort Worth, where I had recently opened a practice. We liked being away from the city, but the hour-plus commute to the office was wearing on me. I had even rented an apartment closer to the office so I wouldn't have to drive home every night and face the possibility of standstill traffic on the Dallas-Fort Worth interstates.

Our kids were not fans of the lake house and always told us, "It's too far to come out and visit!" They had small children, and I didn't blame them for not wanting to get in the car for two hours just to drop by.

In late 2019 the owner of our lake house development began building new homes across the street from us. That meant we would be watching construction for a couple of years, accompanied by the clatter and roar of heavy equipment, and the unhealthy dust in the air and dirt on the roads near us. I didn't want to go through that.

Finally, in January 2020, I said, "This is nuts. Why on earth did I buy this house? I'm going to put it up for sale." I felt certain it was the right decision. When I told Mary, she pressed me to be sure it was not a knee-jerk reaction but was right for the long-term.

"I feel it in my gut," I told her. "Let's see what this place is worth, and maybe we can sell it and find something better."

She agreed, and we were happy to learn that our property had doubled in value in just five years. We put it on the market and it sold quickly, in the first month. In the meantime we were looking at houses near to our son and his family. I had the feeling we needed to be closer to them as well.

One morning while having coffee, I had another urgent gut feeling from the Holy Spirit about a particular house we were going to see.

"This is the one," I told Mary. "I feel it. We need to see it in the next hour or two."

We toured the house that morning and liked it a lot. When we first got there, Mary walked through the door and announced, "This is my house." It had lots of light and windows and the other features we were looking for. It was near my office and right down the street from our son. We made an offer on it that night, and it was accepted. At the same time we put our offer in, someone else was calling to put in an offer. We beat them with our offer by only seconds.

In that same month, February, our lake house sold, and we bought the new house, closing on it on March 1. We moved in a few days later. A week after that, on around March 11, the COVID-19 crisis hit hard, and the real estate market shut down. Had we waited even a few days, we couldn't have even gotten movers. We would have been stuck in the lake house, far from family, waiting out the pandemic.

People have since asked me, How on earth did you time it so well? The answer is, I didn't. It was the Holy Spirit. His timing is perfect. He pushed us to sell one house, gave us the money we needed to make a move to a better location, and did it all within days of a pandemic that caused America to grind to a stop. As a result of the move, our kids and grandkids were nearby, and we could go over to their house on our golf cart or bikes during the quarantine. The grandkids could visit us on their bikes as well.

Having us nearby gave them a sense of security and safety. We felt incredibly blessed and loved by how the Lord moved us to the right place at just the right time.

GUIDANCE IN THE STORMS

We all are going to need that kind of leadership from the Holy Spirit in the days to come. COVID-19 and other pandemics are merely the beginning of what the Bible says the future holds. Revelation 6 tells of a plague that will kill one-fourth of mankind. Imagine an illness so powerful and so sweeping that one out of every four humans perishes! Now imagine the Holy Spirit giving you specific guidance to prepare you for it and put you in the right place. There will surely come a day when hearing and responding to His voice is a matter of life and death. Now is the time for us to get better at both!

Isaiah the Old Testament prophet wrote of difficult events coming on the earth, and the proper response of the faithful, saying:

> Go, my people, enter your rooms and shut the doors behind you; hide yourselves for a little while until his wrath has passed by. See, the LORD is coming out of his dwelling to punish the people of the earth for their sins. The earth will disclose the blood shed on it; the earth will conceal its slain no longer.
>
> —ISAIAH 26:20–21, NIV

It's as if he foresaw what the world would look like during pandemics and plagues, and he counseled prudence.

In 1986 David Wilkerson gave my friend Mike Evans an incredible prophecy: "I see a plague coming on the world, and the bars and churches and government will shut down. The plague will hit New York City and shake it like it has never been shaken. The plague is going to force prayerless Believers into radical prayer and into their Bibles, and repentance will be the cry from the man of God in the pulpit. And out of it will come a third Great Awakening that will sweep America and the world." Mike has written a book, *A Great Awakening Is Coming!*, to share how God is working to stir revival in the hearts of people during a time of struggle and offer hope that the Lord has not left us, but is preparing us for a coming Great Awakening.[1]

Well-known prophetic minister John Paul Jackson, who is now with the Lord, was emphatic about what he dubbed "the perfect storm" the world is headed for. He called it God's loving chastening because "The church has to become a living light again," he said on a video teaching. "The church has to become…a change agent in this earth, especially a change agent in this nation."[2]

Jackson identified five elements of this perfect storm: religion, politics, economics, war, and geophysical events, which include plagues. "Massive problems in these five areas will come often and in combination, and sometimes repeatedly," he said. "Different areas of the United States will experience different severities….It's the combination and the rapidity that will make the storm problematic….This storm will not be short-lived. It will come in waves, one after another….There will be an epidemic that will take many lives, and it will not just be here in the United States but it will also be here and elsewhere. It might actually begin elsewhere and come in here."[3] I find it interesting that during the COVID-19 lockdown, tornadoes tore through the South, doing great damage.

Jackson believed that "this storm is coming because the church, the body of Christ, really is no longer the backbone of this nation….Whenever we sin, it causes God's hand to lift. To the degree God's hand lifts, the enemy has a chance to come in. And right now, God's hand is lifting off this country."[4]

Jackson was not the only one who saw pandemics as messages from God to the church and the nations. During the COVID-19 pandemic Anne Graham Lotz, the daughter of the late evangelist Billy Graham, said there may be a "blessing in the coronavirus" and that God might be using the pandemic "to get our attention so that we will listen to His message." She proposed that this might spark a "national spiritual renewal."[5]

"It's time to pray!" she wrote on her blog. "It's time to turn away from our sin, self-centeredness and secularism, and turn to God in faith and trust.... If we heed God's message, He can calm the storm and bring us through to a time of spiritual revival and national renewal," she said.[6]

She also quoted 2 Chronicles 7:13–15 (NIV), where the Lord says, "When I shut up the heavens so there is no rain, or command locusts to devour the land or send a plague among my people, if my people, who are called by my name, will humble themselves and pray and seek my face and turn from their wicked ways, then I will hear from heaven, and I will forgive their sin and will heal their land. Now My eyes will be open and my ears attentive to the prayers offered."[7]

"Could the silver lining in the black cloud of the coronavirus be this?" asked Graham. "That it causes America to look up and listen to what God has to say, and therefore becomes the trigger for a national spiritual revival? May it be so!"[8]

Graham also discussed how God came to Moses in a "dense cloud," when the Israelites were camped at the base of Mount Sinai (Exod. 19:9). She wrote, "During this time, God spoke to me through His Word: Anne, even though you walk through the valley of the shadow of death, you will fear no evil; for I am with you.... So, do not fear, for I am with you, do not be dismayed, for I am your God. I will strengthen you and help you; I will uphold you with My righteous right hand."[9]

Many voices were affirming this same thing. Chuck Pierce, a well-established prophetic minister, says that God told him in September 2019, months before the appearance of COVID-19, that the "nations would come into turmoil until Passover," which in 2020 was April 8–16. On January 26, 2020, Pierce gave a prophetic word that a "massive plague-like invasion...would test us through Passover."[10] Cindy Jacobs gave a similar prophecy to Chuck's a few weeks before that regarding the first three months of 2020, and told Chuck that he should be cautious about how much he travels. Chuck related this conversation:

"I had gone 570,000 miles last year and was weary from all the travel and warfare. She [Cindy] actually shared that the Lord was saying that I needed rest, but I recognized the admonition to be a caution on my travel for the first three months of 2020. Therefore, I have watched the Lord make sure I've had more time to rest and write, and have actually stopped most international travel during these three months."[11]

Pierce emphasized two passages in the Book of Joel as prophetic for this hour:

> Do not be afraid, land; exult and rejoice, for the LORD has done great things! Do not be afraid, beasts of the field, because the wild pastures flourish, because the tree bears its fruit; the fig tree and the vine yield their abundance. And children of Zion, exult and rejoice in the LORD your God, because He has given to you the early rain for vindication. He showers down rains for you, the early rain and the latter rain, as before.
>
> —JOEL 2:21–23, MEV

> Hurry and come, all you surrounding nations, and gather there. Bring down Your warriors, O LORD. Let the nations

> be roused, and go up to the Valley of Jehoshaphat; for there I
> will sit to judge all the surrounding nations....Multitudes,
> multitudes, in the valley of decision! For the day of the
> LORD is near in the valley of the decision.
>
> —JOEL 3:11–12, 14, MEV

No prophetic person has the entire picture, but God certainly
warns and gives insight to His body through people who hear His
voice. It is vitally important that we listen to what prophetic and
wise people are saying about upcoming pandemics and other world
events. Media and governments may give us facts, but only hearing
what God is saying can give insight from heaven.

This insight comes not just from prophets and ministers, but to
each one of us. Every believer is equipped to hear from God! Jesus
said in John 16:13 that the Holy Spirit will guide believers into
all truth and tell us what the future holds. This is a life-changing
promise that each of us needs to walk in for ourselves. It is time to
hear from God in our own hearts, and to listen as well to what He
is saying through others. Only then will we act and react rightly
during pandemics and other crises.

Ultimately God plans to wipe out all diseases, plagues, and pandemics. His goal is the healing of all humanity. The prophet Isaiah
spoke of God's good intent when he wrote:

> "I have seen their ways, but I will heal them; I will guide
> them and restore comfort to Israel's mourners, creating
> praise on their lips. Peace, peace, to those far and near,"
> says the LORD. "And I will heal them."
>
> —ISAIAH 57:18–19, NIV

Maybe you don't have a personal relationship with God's Son,
Jesus Christ, yet. You need to know that He wants to make you

whole in your body, mind, and spirit. He has a plan to protect you from pandemics, and to give you life more abundantly. He is your shield and very great reward—and He will be your best friend like He is mine.

If you haven't met my best friend, Jesus, I would like to take this opportunity to introduce Him to you. It is very simple. If you are ready to let Him come into your life and become your best friend, all you need to do is sincerely pray this prayer:

> *Lord Jesus, I want to know You as my Savior and Lord. I believe You are the Son of God and that You died for my sins. I also believe You were raised from the dead and now sit at the right hand of the Father praying for me. I ask You to forgive me for my sins and change my heart so that I can be Your child and live with You eternally. Thank You for Your peace. Help me to walk with You so that I can begin to know You as my best friend and my Lord. Amen.*

If you have prayed this prayer, you have just made the most important decision of your life. I rejoice with you in your decision and your new relationship with Jesus. Please contact my publisher at pray4me@charismamedia.com so that we can send you some materials that will help you become established in your relationship with the Lord. We look forward to hearing from you.

SAMPLE MENUS FOR A HEALTHY GUT
DAY 1

Breakfast

1–2 eggs scrambled or over-easy, cooked in avocado oil
Half or quarter of an avocado
Piece of toasted millet bread with olive oil (not butter) on top
¼ cup of berries

Lunch

Big salad with lots of olive oil (2–4 tablespoons)
Onions
Feta cheese (not too much)
Cucumbers
Tomatoes
Mushrooms
3–4 ounces grilled chicken breast, cut into chunks and sautéed
with onion

Dinner

3–4 ounces of grilled or baked chicken breast, turkey breast,
salmon, wild shrimp scampi, or lean filet of beef once or
twice a week. Avoid processed meats. Go with organic
grass-fed meats, nothing processed.
Sweet potato, medium
Green vegetables (broccoli, asparagus, cabbage), as much as
desired
2–3 tablespoons Greek olive oil on a salad of romaine, arugula,
and field greens, with cucumbers, tomatoes, carrots, onions,
and a small amount of feta cheese

DAY 2

Breakfast

Steel-cut oatmeal

½ cup low-fat, low-sugar coconut or almond milk, or water (I
combine these overnight and put it in the fridge. The next
morning it's easier to cook. Just add more water, almond
milk, or coconut milk.)

After cooking I add the following:

Stevia or monk fruit or erythritol

Pecans or walnuts

¼ cup berries, which I smoosh into the oatmeal

Lunch

Chicken salad with avocado oil mayonnaise

Onions

Celery

Feta cheese

Pickle

Optional: make this a sandwich with a piece of millet bread or a
wrap with a romaine lettuce leaf

Dinner

Soup with an organic beef or chicken broth, bone broth, or
curry base

Broccoli, as much as desired

Onions, as much as desired

Mushrooms, as much as desired

Other green vegetables, as much as desired

One of the meats listed for the Day 1 dinner (3–4 ounces per
person)

Basmati rice (the size of a tennis ball per person)
Garlic or cilantro (the key ingredients for delicious chicken
    soup)
2–3 tablespoons olive oil per serving (add after boiling the
    soup)

As a general practice, boil the meat, brown it in a skillet on low to medium heat, or put it in a slow cooker or multi-cooker, then add it to a soup with onion, broccoli, basmati rice, garlic, and cilantro if you like. After boiling, add olive oil.

Try wild shrimp scampi with low-fat, low-sugar coconut milk, and cook it with avocado oil, not butter. I use it in soups with chicken stock and onions and perhaps garlic. Flavor it with peppers to taste.

Your body craves a simple lifestyle and menu—and it's easy to train your appetite to enjoy these things!

APPENDIX B

RECOMMENDED NUTRITIONAL PRODUCTS
DIVINE HEALTH PRODUCTS

964 International Parkway, Suite 1630
Lake Mary, Florida 32746
Phone: (407)732-6952
Website: www.drcolbert.com
Email: info@drcolbert.com

- Green Supremefood: Ten certified USDA organic fermented vegetables and six fermented grasses (including wheatgrass, barley grass, alfalfa grass, spirulina, and chlorella), with prebiotics, probiotics, fiber, and enzymes. In apple cinnamon flavor.

- Red Supremefood: Nine certified USDA organic fruits with probiotics, prebiotics, and fiber. Delicious flavor.

- Ketozone Fiber: Delicious flavored fiber with prebiotics that support gut health.

- Beyond Biotics: My favorite probiotic and the one I place most of my patients on.

- Enhanced Multivitamin: Take one in the morning (active forms of individual vitamins and chelated minerals).

- Glutathione-Boosting Supplements:

1. NAC-N Acetyl Cysteine—500 mg twice a day (from health food store)

2. Cellgevity (Dr. Colbert's favorite Glutathione Booster)—take 2 twice a day or MaxOne—take 1 capsule twice a day. To order: 1.801.316.6380 and use code 231599.

HOW TO PROPERLY WASH YOUR HANDS[1]

Rinse first

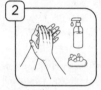

Lather soap

Rub palms

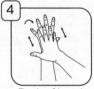

Back of hands

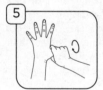

Base of thumbs

Between fingers

Around wrists

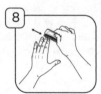

Under fingernails

Rinse & dry

NOTES

INTRODUCTION

1. John M. Barry, *The Great Influenza* (New York: Penguin Books, 2005), 276, https://archive.org/details/greatinfluenzaep00barr/page/276/mode/2up.
2. Barry, *The Great Influenza*, 326.
3. Barry, *The Great Influenza*, 237, 246.
4. Barry, *The Great Influenza*, photos 14 and 21.

CHAPTER 1

1. *The Oxford English Dictionary*, s.v. "influenza," accessed May 3, 2020, https://archive.org/details/oxfordenglishdic0007unse/page/940/mode/2up.
2. "'Tis the (Flu) Season: The History of 'Influenza,'" Merriam-Webster, December 16, 2019, https://www.merriam-webster.com/words-at-play/influenza-flu-word-history-origin.
3. Barry, *The Great Influenza*, 101–3, 451.
4. Elinor Levy and Tom Monte, *The Ten Best Tools to Boost Your Immune System* (Boston: Houghton Mifflin, 1997), 23, https://archive.org/details/tenbesttoolstobo00levy/page/n5/mode/2up; Craig Freudenrich and Patrick J. Kiger, "How Viruses Work," HowStuffWorks, accessed May 3, 2020, https://science.howstuffworks.com/life/cellular-microscopic/virus-human2.htm.
5. Levy and Monte, *The Ten Best Tools to Boost Your Immune System*, 24–25.
6. "Disease Burden of Influenza," Centers for Disease Control and Prevention, last reviewed April 17, 2020, https://www.cdc.gov/flu/about/burden/index.html; "Global Influenza Strategy 2019–2030," World Health Organization, accessed May 3, 2020, https://www.who.int/influenza/Global_Influenza_Strategy_2019_2030_Summary_English.pdf?ua=1.
7. Quentin Fottrell, "'The Attack Rate Is Relatively High as There's No Immunity to It.' Why Coronavirus Was Never Going to Be Just Another Flu," MarketWatch, March 31, 2020, https://www.marketwatch.com/story/coronavirus-vs-the-flu-its-just-like-other-viruses-and-we-should-go-about-our-normal-business-right-wrong-heres-why-2020-03-09.

8. Edwin D. Kilbourne, "Influenza Pandemics of the 20th Century," *Emerging Infectious Diseases* 12, no. 1 (January 2006): 9–14, https:doi.org/10.3201/eid1201.051254.

9. Joel Fuhrman, *Super Immunity: The Essential Nutrition Guide for Boosting Your Body's Defenses to Live Longer, Stronger, and Disease Free* (New York: HarperCollins, 2011), 3, https://www.amazon.com/Super-Immunity-Essential-Nutrition-Boosting/dp/0062080644.

10. Fuhrman, *Super Immunity*, 4.

11. Dave Roos, "How Five of History's Worst Pandemics Finally Ended," History.com, updated March 27, 2020, https://www.history.com/news/pandemics-end-plague-cholera-black-death-smallpox.

12. Roos, "How Five of History's Worst Pandemics Finally Ended."

13. "History of Quarantine," Centers for Disease Control and Prevention, accessed May 3, 2020, https://www.cdc.gov/quarantine/historyquarantine.html.

14. Roos, "How Five of History's Worst Pandemics Finally Ended."

15. Annalee Newitz, "What Social Distancing Looked Like in 1666," New York Times, March 29, 2020, https://www.nytimes.com/2020/03/29/opinion/covid-plague-samuel-pepys.html.

16. Newitz, "What Social Distancing Looked Like in 1666."

17. Jesse Greenspan, "The Rise and Fall of Smallpox," History.com, updated August 22, 2018, https://www.history.com/news/the-rise-and-fall-of-smallpox.

18. "Smallpox: Signs and Symptoms," Centers for Disease Control and Prevention, accessed May 3, 2020, https://www.cdc.gov/smallpox/symptoms/index.html.

19. Roos, "How Five of History's Worst Pandemics Finally Ended."

20. "Smallpox," Centers for Disease Control and Prevention.

21. Kathleen Tuthill, "John Snow and the Broad Street Pump: On the Trail of an Epidemic," Cricket 31, no. 3 (November 2003): 23–31, https://www.ph.ucla.edu/epi/snow/snowcricketarticle.html.

22. Roos, "How Five of History's Worst Pandemics Finally Ended."

23. Tuthill, "John Snow and the Broad Street Pump."

24. Tuthill, "John Snow and the Broad Street Pump."

25. Barry, *The Great Influenza*, 4–5.

26. Barry, The Great Influenza, photo 10.

27. Barry, *The Great Influenza*, 238.
28. Fuhrman, *Super Immunity*, 35–36.
29. Barry, *The Great Influenza*, 371.
30. Owen Jarus, "Twenty of the Worst Epidemics and Pandemics in History," Live Science, March 20, 2020, https://www.livescience.com/worst-epidemics-and-pandemics-in-history.html.
31. "Deadliest Pandemics of the 20th Century," CNN, April 27, 2009, https://www.cnn.com/2009/HEALTH/04/27/pandemics.history/index.html.
32. "Deadliest Pandemics of the 20th Century," CNN.
33. Barry, *The Great Influenza*, 114.
34. Jarus, "Twenty of the Worst Epidemics and Pandemics in History."
35. "Past Pandemics," World Health Organization, accessed May 3, 2020, http://www.euro.who.int/en/health-topics/communicable-diseases/influenza/pandemic-influenza/past-pandemics.
36. "Deadliest Pandemics of the 20th Century," CNN.
37. Jarus, "Twenty of the Worst Epidemics and Pandemics in History."
38. "Consensus Document on the Epidemiology of Severe Acute Respiratory Syndrome (SARS)," World Health Organization, May 2003, who.int/csr/sars/en/WHOconsensus.pdf.
39. "2014–2016 Ebola Outbreak in West Africa," Centers for Disease Control and Prevention, last reviewed March 8, 2019, https://www.cdc.gov/vhf/ebola/history/2014-2016-outbreak/index.html.
40. "Zika Virus: Overview," Centers for Disease Control and Prevention, last reviewed October 7, 2019, https://www.cdc.gov/zika/about/overview.html; "Zika Virus: Zika in the US," Centers for Disease Control and Prevention, last reviewed November 7, 2019, https://www.cdc.gov/zika/geo/index.html.
41. "Disease Burden of Influenza," Centers for Disease Control and Prevention, last reviewed April 17, 2020, https://www.cdc.gov/flu/about/burden/index.html.
42. Erika Edwards, "Not Just Older People: Younger Adults Are Also Getting the Coronavirus," NBC Universal, March 17, 2020, https://www.nbcnews.com/health/health-news/not-just-older-people-younger-adults-are-also-getting-coronavirus-n1160416.
43. Mike Stobbe, "Study: COVID-19 Can Be Spread by People Who Are Showing No Symptoms," The Columbian, April 1, 2020, https://www.columbian.com/news/2020/apr/01/

study-covid-19-can-be-spread-by-people-who-are-showing-no-symptoms/.

44. "White House Projects Grim Toll From Coronavirus," New York Times, updated April 7, 2020, https://www.nytimes.com/2020/03/31/world/coronavirus-live-news-updates.html.

45. Jiao Zhao et al., "Relationship Between the ABO Blood Group and the COVID-19 Susceptibility," MedRxiv, March 27, 2020, https://doi.org/10.1101/2020.03.11.20031096.

46. Nell Greenfieldboyce, "The New Coronavirus Appears to Take a Greater Toll on Men Than on Women," NPR, April 10, 2020, https://www.npr.org/sections/goatsandsoda/2020/04/10/831883664/the-new-coronavirus-appears-to-take-a-greater-toll-on-men-than-on-women.

47. Holly Secon, "People Can Get the Coronavirus More Than Once, Experts Warn—Recovering Does Not Necessarily Make You Immune," Business Insider, February 27, 2020, https://www.businessinsider.com/wuhan-coronavirus-risk-of-reinfection-2020-2?op=1.

48. "Past Pandemics," World Health Organization.

49. Fuhrman, *Super Immunity*, 8.

CHAPTER 2

1. Levy and Monte, *The Ten Best Tools to Boost Your Immune System*, 9–10.

2. Barry, *The Great Influenza*, 107.

3. Barry, *The Great Influenza*, 108.

4. Levy and Monte, *The Ten Best Tools to Boost Your Immune System*, 11–12.

5. Levy and Monte, *The Ten Best Tools to Boost Your Immune System*, 13–14, 23.

6. Levy and Monte, *The Ten Best Tools to Boost Your Immune System*, 14–17.

7. Levy and Monte, *The Ten Best Tools to Boost Your Immune System*, 21–22.

8. Levy and Monte, *The Ten Best Tools to Boost Your Immune System*, 22.

9. Roos, "How Five of History's Worst Pandemics Finally Ended."

CHAPTER 3

1. Robynne Chutkan, *The Microbiome Solution: A Radical New Way to Heal Your Body From the Inside Out* (New York: Avery, 2015), 3, https://books.google.com/books?id=UIYVBgAAQBAJ&q.

2. National Institutes of Health, "NIH Human Microbiome Project Defines Normal Bacterial Makeup of the Body," news release, June 13, 2012, https://www.nih.gov/news-events/news-releases/nih-human-microbiome-project-defines-normal-bacterial-makeup-body.

3. Chutkan, *The Microbiome Solution*, 14.

4. Yasmine Belkaid and Timothy W. Hand, "Role of the Microbiota in Immunity and Inflammation," *Cell* 157, no. 1 (March 27, 2014): 121–41, https://doi.org/10.1016/j.cell.2014.03.011.

5. Giulia Enders, *Gut: The Inside Story of Our Body's Most Underrated Organ* (Vancouver, Canada: Greystone, 2015), 148, https://archive.org/details/gutinsidestoryof0000ende/page/148/mode/2up.

6. Belkaid and Hand, "Role of the Microbiota in Immunity and Inflammation."

7. David Perlmutter with Kristin Loberg, *Brain Maker: The Power of Gut Microbes to Heal and Protect Your Brain—for Life* (London: Yellow Kite, 2015), 7, https://www.amazon.com/Brain-Maker-Power-Microbes-Protect/dp/1478985550.

8. Fuhrman, *Super Immunity*, 34.

9. Belkaid and Hand, "Role of the Microbiota in Immunity and Inflammation."

10. Fuhrman, *Super Immunity*, 32–33.

11. Fuhrman, *Super Immunity*, 15, 35.

12. Perlmutter and Loberg, *Brain Maker*, 149–53.

13. For more information, refer to my book *Dr. Colbert's Healthy Gut Zone* in January 2021 and beyond.

14. Albert Sanchez et al., "Role of Sugars in Human Neutrophilic Phagocytosis," *The American Journal of Clinical Nutrition* 26, no. 11 (November 1973): 1180–84, https://doi.org/10.1093/ajcn/26.11.1180.

15. Atli Arnarson, "A1 vs. A2 Milk—Does It Matter?," Healthline, March 14, 2019, https://www.healthline.com/nutrition/a1-vs-a2-milk.

16. Perlmutter and Loberg, *Brain Maker*, 56–59.

17. I am writing a book about this, called *Dr. Colbert's Healthy Gut Zone Diet*, which I consider a partner to this book; I encourage you to read it for more information about keeping a healthy gut.

18. Fuhrman, *Super Immunity*, 69.

19. Fuhrman, *Super Immunity*, 62–63, 65.

20. Fuhrman, *Super Immunity*, 118.

21. Hong Zhang et al., "Prospective Study of Probiotic Supplementation Results in Immune Stimulation and Improvement of Upper Respiratory Infection Rate," *Synthetic and Systems Biotechnology* 3, no. 2 (March 12, 2018): 113–20, https://doi.org/10.1016/j.synbio.2018.03.001.

22. Hrefna Palsdottir, "11 Probiotic Foods That Are Super Healthy," Healthline, August 28, 2018, https://www.healthline.com/nutrition/11-super-healthy-probiotic-foods.

23. Enders, *Gut*, 248–50.

24. Raphael Kellman, *The Microbiome Breakthrough: Harness the Power of Your Gut Bacteria to Boost Your Mood and Heal Your Body* (New York: Da Capo Press, 2018), 112, https://www.amazon.com/Microbiome-Breakthrough-Harness-Power-Bacteria/dp/0738284602.

25. Arlene Semeco, "The 19 Best Prebiotic Foods You Should Eat," Healthline, June 8, 2016, https://www.healthline.com/nutrition/19-best-prebiotic-foods.

26. Chutkan, *The Microbiome Solution*, 125.

27. Fuhrman, *Super Immunity*, 111.

28. Fuhrman, *Super Immunity*, 112.

29. Fuhrman, *Super Immunity*, 69–70.

30. Norbert D. Weber et al., "*In Vitro* Virucidal Effects of *Allium sativum* (Garlic) Extract and Compounds," *Planta Medica* 58, no. 5 (1992): 417–23, https:doi.org/10.1055/s-2006-961504.

CHAPTER 4

1. Luciana Besedovsky, Tanja Lange, and Jan Born, "Sleep and Immune Function," *Pflügers Archiv* 463, no. 1 (January 2012): 121–37, https:doi.org/10.1007/s00424-011-1044-0.

2. Najib T. Ayas et al., "A Prospective Study of Sleep Duration and Coronary Heart Disease in Women," *Archives of Internal Medicine* 163, no. 2 (2003): 205–9, https://doi.org/10.1001/archinte.163.2.205.

3. "Get Sleep: Judgment and Safety," Harvard Medical School, last reviewed December 16, 2008, http://healthysleep.med.harvard.edu/need-sleep/whats-in-it-for-you/judgment-safety. See also A. Williamson and A. Feyer, "Moderate Sleep Deprivation Produces Impairments in Cognitive and Motor Performance Equivalent to Legally Prescribed Levels of Alcohol Intoxication," *Occupational and Environmental Medicine* 57, no. 10 (October 2000): 649–55, https://doi.org/10.1136/oem.57.10.649.

4. "How Much Sleep Do We Really Need?," SleepFoundation.org, accessed May 3, 2020, https://www.sleepfoundation.org/articles/how-much-sleep-do-we-really-need.

5. "Sleep Apnea," Mayo Clinic, accessed May 3, 2020, https://www.mayoclinic.org/diseases-conditions/sleep-apnea/symptoms-causes/syc-20377631.

6. Irina V. Zhdanova et al., "Sleep-Inducing Effects of Low Doses of Melatonin Ingested in the Evening," *Clinical Pharmacology and Therapeutics* 57, no. 5 (May 1995): 552–58, https:doi.org/10.1016/0009-9236(95)90040-3.

CHAPTER 5

1. Suzanne C. Segerstrom and Gregory E. Miller, "Psychological Stress and the Human Immune System: A Meta-Analytic Study of 30 Years of Inquiry," *Psychological Bulletin* 130, no. 4 (July 2004): 601–30, https:doi.org/10.1037/0033-2909.130.4.601.

2. Jennifer N. Morey et al., "Current Directions in Stress and Human Immune Function," *Current Opinion in Psychology* 5 (October 1, 2015): 13–17, https://doi.org/10.1016/j.copsyc.2015.03.007.

3. Thomas G. Allison et al., "Medical and Economic Costs of Psychologic Distress in Patients With Coronary Artery Disease," *Mayo Clinic Proceedings* 70, no. 8 (August 1995): 734–42, https://doi.org/10.4065/70.8.734.

4. Hans Selye, "A Syndrome Produced by Diverse Nocuous Agents," *Nature* 138 (July 4, 1936): 32, https://doi.org/10.1038/138032a0.

5. M. Irwin et al., "Reduction of Immune Function in Life Stress and Depression," *Biological Psychiatry* 27, no. 1 (January 1, 1990): 22–30, https://doi.org/10.1016/0006-3223(90)90016-u.

6. S. Kennedy, "Immunological Consequences of Acute and Chronic Stressors: Mediating Role of Interpersonal Relationships," *British*

   Journal of Medical Psychology 61, no. 1 (March 1988): 77–85,
   https://doi.org/10.1111/j.2044-8341.1988.tb02766.x.

7.   David D. Burns, *Feeling Good: The New Mood Therapy*
      (New York: Signet, 1980), https://archive.org/details/
      feelinggoodnewmo00burn_0/page/40/mode/2up.

8.   Robert A. Emmons, *Thanks! How the New Science of Gratitude Can
      Make You Happier* (Boston: Houghton Mifflin, 2007), 12, https://
      archive.org/details/thankshownewscie00emmo/page/n5/mode/2up;
      Deborah D. Danner, David A. Snowdon, and Wallace V. Friesen,
      "Positive Emotions in Early Life and Longevity: Findings From the
      Nun Study," *Journal of Personality and Social Psychology* 80, no. 5
      (May 2001): 804–13, https://doi.org/10.1037/0022-3514.80.5.804.

9.   Doc Childre and Howard Martin with Donna Beech, *The
      HeartMath Solution* (New York: HarperCollins, 1999), https://
      archive.org/details/heartmathsolutio00docl/page/n5/mode/2up.

10. Childre, Martin, and Beech, *The HeartMath Solution*; Doc Lew
      Childre, *Freeze-Frame: Fast Action Stress Relief* (Boulder Creek,
      CA: Planetary Publications, 1994), https://archive.org/details/
      freezeframefasta00chil/page/n7/mode/2up.

11. Winston Churchill, "We Shall Fight on the Beaches" (speech,
      House of Commons, London, June 4, 1940), https://
      winstonchurchill.org/resources/speeches/1940-the-finest-hour/
      we-shall-fight-on-the-beaches/.

CHAPTER 6

1.   Josh Barney, "Exercise May Protect Against Deadly COVID-19
      Complication, Research Suggests," UVA Today, April 15, 2020,
      https://news.virginia.edu/content/exercise-may-protect-against-
      deadly-covid-19-complication-research-suggests.

2.   Ruth Sander, "Exercise Boosts Immune Response," *Nursing Older
      People* 24, no. 6 (June 29, 2012): 11, https://doi.org/10.7748/
      nop.24.6.11.s11.

3.   James A. Blumenthal et al., "Effects of Exercise Training on Older
      Patients With Major Depression," *Archives of Internal Medicine*
      159, no. 19 (October 25, 1999): 2349–56, https://doi.org/10.1001/
      archinte.159.19.2349.

4.   Meir J. Stampfer et al., "Primary Prevention of Coronary Heart
      Disease in Women Through Diet and Lifestyle," *New England*

Journal of Medicine 343 (July 6, 2000): 16–22, https://doi. org/10.1056/NEJM200007063430103.

5. Wanda Pilch et al., "Effect of a Single Finnish Sauna Session on White Blood Cell Profile and Cortisol Levels in Athletes and Non-Athletes," *Journal of Human Kinetics* 39, no. 1 (December 18, 2013): 127–35, https://doi.org/10.2478/hukin-2013-0075. See also B. Dugué and E. Leppänen, "Adaptation Related to Cytokines in Man: Effects of Regular Swimming in Ice-Cold Water," *Clinical Physiology* 20, no. 2 (March 2000): 114–21, https://doi.org/10.1046/ j.1365-2281.2000.00235.x; E. Ernst et al., "Regular Sauna Bathing and the Incidence of Common Colds," *Annals of Medicine* 22, no. 4 (1990): 225–27, https://doi.org/10.3109/07853899009148930; B. Dugué, E. Leppänen, and R. Gräsbeck, "Effects of Thermal Stress (Sauna + Swimming in Ice-Cold Water) in Man on the Blood Concentration and Production of Pro-Inflammatory Cytokines and Stress Hormones," *Pathophysiology* 5, suppl. 1 (June 1998): 149, https://doi.org/10.1016/S0928-4680(98)80866-3; Baris E. Dayanc et al., "Dissecting the Role of Hyperthermia in Natural Killer Cell Mediated Anti-Tumor Responses," *International Journal of Hyperthermia* 24, no. 1 (February 2008): 41–56, https://doi. org/10.1080/02656730701858297.

CHAPTER 7

1. Michael Murray, "Coronavirus, Precautions, and Strengthening the Immune System," *iHerb* (blog), January 29, 2020, https://www. iherb.com/blog/coronavirus-precautions-and-strengthening-the-immune-system/897.

2. "Thymosin," Holistic Solutions, accessed May 4, 2020, https:// holisticsolutionsdoc.com/thymosin/.

3. Kathy Maupin and Brett Newcomb, "Thymosin Alpha (TA1)—A New Cancer Treatment," BioBalance Health, February 24, 2020, https://www.biobalancehealth.com/thymosin-alpha-ta1-a-new-cancer-treatment.

4. Maupin and Newcomb, "Thymosin Alpha (TA1)—A New Cancer Treatment."

5. Rebecca Gillaspy, "What Are Cytokines?—Definition, Types, and Function," Study.com, accessed May 4, 2020, https://study.com/ academy/lesson/what-are-cytokines-definition-types-function.html.

6. NCI Dictionary of Cancer Terms, s.v. "cytokine storm," accessed May 4, 2020, https://www.cancer.gov/publications/dictionaries/cancer-terms/def/797584.

7. Barry, *The Great Influenza*, 187.

8. Barry, *The Great Influenza*, 245.

9. Barry, *The Great Influenza*, 190.

10. Teresa Richter, "Thymosin Alpha-1," Kirkland Natural Medicine, March 31, 2020, https://drteresarichter.com/blog/thymosin-alpha-1.

11. Radhia Gleis, "Dr. Cannell and the Curious Case of the Flu," Advanced Health Institute, June 7, 2019, https://www.advancedhealthinstitute.com/single-post/2019/06/07/Dr-Cannell-and-the-Curious-Case-of-the-Flu.

12. Adrian R. Martineau et al., "Vitamin D Supplementation to Prevent Acute Respiratory Tract Infections: Systematic Review and Meta-Analysis of Individual Participant Data," *BMJ* 356 (February 15, 2017), https://doi.org/10.1136/bmj.i6583.

13. Fuhrman, *Super Immunity*, 104. See also J. J. Cannell et al., "Epidemic Influenza and Vitamin D," *Epidemiology and Infection* 134, no. 6 (December 2006): 1129–40, https://doi.org/10.1017/S0950268806007175; Alexandra V. Yamshchikov et al., "Vitamin D for Treatment and Prevention of Infectious Diseases: A Systematic Review of Randomized Controlled Trials," *Endocrine Practice* 15, no. 5 (July 2009): 438–49, https://doi.org/10.4158/EP09101.ORR.

14. James R. Sabetta et al., "Serum 25-Hydroxyvitamin D and the Incidence of Acute Viral Respiratory Tract Infections in Healthy Adults," *PLOS One* 5, no. 6 (June 14, 2010): e11088, https://doi.org/10.1371/journal.pone.0011088.

15. Gleis, "Dr. Cannell and the Curious Case of the Flu."

16. Murray, "Coronavirus, Precautions, and Strengthening the Immune System."

17. Mike McRae, "COVID-19 Deaths Are Being Linked to Vitamin D Deficiency. Here's What That Means," Science Alert, May 1, 2020, https://www.sciencealert.com/covid-deaths-are-being-linked-with-vitamin-d-deficiency-here-s-what-that-means.

18. Ohio State University, "Zinc Helps Against Infection by Tapping Brakes in Immune Response," ScienceDaily, February 7, 2013, www.sciencedaily.com/releases/2013/02/130207131344.htm.

19. Ohio State University. "Zinc Helps Against Infection by Tapping Brakes in Immune Response." See also Ming-Jie Liu et al., "ZIP8 Regulates Host Defense Through Zinc-Mediated Inhibition of NF-kB," *Cell Reports* 3, no. 2 (February 21, 2013): P386–400, https://doi.org/10.1016/j.celrep.2013.01.009.

20. Fuhrman, *Super Immunity*, 103.

21. Fuhrman, *Super Immunity*, 102.

22. Ohio State University, "Zinc Helps Against Infection by Tapping Brakes in Immune Response."

23. "Fight Flu and Cold Season With Five Liposomal Powerhouses," QuickSilver Scientific, February 18, 2019, https://www.quicksilverscientific.com/blog/fight-flu-and-cold-season-with-five-liposomal-powerhouses/. See also A. Fraternale, S. Brundu, and M. Magnani, "Glutathione and Glutathione Derivatives in Immunotherapy," *Biological Chemistry* 398 no. 2 (February 1, 2017): 261–75, https://doi.org/10.1515/hsz-2016-0202.

24. Tasreen Alibhai, "Support Your Immune System This Cold and Flu Season with Glutathione," Vitalia Naturopathic Doctors, accessed May 4, 2020, https://vitaliahealthcare.ca/blog/glutathione-support-for-the-flu-season/.

25. S. De Flora, C. Grassi, and L. Carati, "Attenuation of Influenza-Like Symptomatology and Improvement of Cell-Mediated Immunity With Long-Term N-Acetylcysteine Treatment," *European Respiratory Journal* 10, no. 7 (July 1997): 1535–41, https://doi.org/10.1183/09031936.97.10071535.

26. J. Cai et al., "Inhibition of Influenza Infection by Glutathione," *Free Radical Biology & Medicine* 34, no. 7 (April 1, 2003): 928–36, https://doi.org/10.1016/s0891-5849(03)00023-6.

27. R. Sinha et al., "Oral Supplementation With Liposomal Glutathione Elevates Body Stores of Glutathione and Markers of Immune Function," *European Journal of Clinical Nutrition* 72, no. 1 (January 2018): 105–11, https://doi.org/10.1038/ejcn.2017.132.

28. "How to Avoid Flu Naturally (and Why Optimized Glutathione Is Important)," ImmuneHealthScience.com, accessed May 4, 2020, http://www.immunehealthscience.com/avoid-flu.html.

29. I. Jaspers et al., "Selenium Deficiency Alters Epithelial Cell Morphology and Responses to Influenza," *Free Radical Biology*

& *Medicine* 42, no. 12 (June 15, 2007): 1826–37, https://doi. org/10.1016/j.freeradbiomed.2007.03.017.

30. Peter R. Hoffman and Marla J. Barry, "The Influence of Selenium on Immune Responses," *Molecular Nutrition & Food Research* 52, no. 11 (November 2008): 1273–80, https://doi.org/10.1002/ mnfr.200700330.

31. Hoffman and Barry, "The Influence of Selenium on Immune Responses."

32. Hoffman and Barry, "The Influence of Selenium on Immune Responses."

33. "How to Avoid Flu Naturally," ImmuneHealthScience.com.

34. Katie Adlam, "*Lactobacillus plantarum* and Its Biological Implications," Microbe Wiki, last edited October 26, 2014, https:// microbewiki.kenyon.edu/index.php/Lactobacillus_plantarum_and_ its_biological_implications.

35. Fuhrman, *Super Immunity*, 104.

36. Chris Kilham, "Three All-Natural Flu Fighters," *Prevention*, January 22, 2013, https://www.prevention.com/health/a20440866/ natural-flu-fighting-herbs-and-supplements/.

37. Fuhrman, *Super Immunity*, 105.

38. Kilham, "Three All-Natural Flu Fighters."

39. Harri Hemilä, "Vitamin C and Infections," *Nutrients* 9, no. 4 (April 2017): 339, https://doi.org/10.3390/nu9040339.

40. "Can Vitamin C Prevent a Cold?," Harvard Health, January 2017, https://www.health.harvard.edu/cold-and-flu/can-vitamin-c- prevent-a-cold.

41. J. R. Thorpe, "How Vitamin C Works to Prevent the Flu," Bustle, November 10, 2019, https://www.bustle.com/p/how-vitamin-c- works-to-prevent-the-flu-19300887. See also Hemilä, "Vitamin C and Infections."

42. "Fight Flu and Cold Season With Five Liposomal Powerhouses," QuickSilver Scientific. See also Y. B. Shaik-Dasthagirisaheb et al., "Role of Vitamins D, E and C in Immunity and Inflammation," *Journal of Biological Regulators and Homeostatic Agents* 27, no. 2 (April–June 2013): 291–95, https://www.ncbi.nlm.nih.gov/ pubmed/23830380; R. Anderson, "Ascorbate-Mediated Stimulation of Neutrophil Motility and Lymphocyte Transformation by Inhibition of the Peroxidase/H2O2/Halide System in Vitro and in

Vivo," *American Journal of Clinical Nutrition* 34, no. 9 (September 1981): 1906–11, https://doi.org/10.1093/ajcn/34.9.1906.

43. "Can Vitamin C Prevent a Cold?," Harvard Health.

44. Murray, "Coronavirus, Precautions, and Strengthening the Immune System."

45. Murray, "Coronavirus, Precautions, and Strengthening the Immune System."

46. "Astralagus," Penn State Hershey, last reviewed March 24, 2015, http://pennstatehershey.adam.com/content.aspx?productid=107&pid=33&gid=000223.

47. S. Gupta, K. P. Mishra, and L. Ganju, "Broad-Spectrum Antiviral Properties of Andrographolide," *Archives of Virology* 162, no. 3 (March 2017): 611–23, https://doi.org/10.1007/s00705-016-3166-3.

48. Y. Ding et al., "Andrographolide Inhibits Influenza A Virus-Induced Inflammation in a Murine Model Through NF-κB and JAK-STAT Signaling Pathway," *Microbes and Infection* 19, no. 12 (December 2017): 605–15, https://doi.org/10.1016/j.micinf.2017.08.009.

49. Julian Friedland, "Is Andrographis the Next Big Immune Booster?," New Hope Network, April 23, 2008, https://www.newhope.com/ingredients/andrographis-next-big-immune-booster.

50. Kilham, "Three All-Natural Flu Fighters."

51. "Fight Flu and Cold Season With Five Liposomal Powerhouses," QuickSilver Scientific. See also Irma Lemaire et al., "Stimulation of Interleukin-1 and -6 Production in Alveolar Macrophages by the Neotropical Liana, *Uncaria tomentosa* (Uña de Gato)," *Journal of Ethnopharmacology* 64, no. 2 (February 1, 1999): 109–15, https://doi.org/10.1016/S0378-8741(98)00113-5; Y. Sheng, C. Bryngelsson, and R. W. Pero, "Enhanced DNA Repair, Immune Function and Reduced Toxicity of C-MED-100, a Novel Aqueous Extract From Uncaria Tomentosa," *Journal of Ethnopharmacology* 69, no. 2 (February 2000): 115–26, https://doi.org/10.1016/s0378-8741(99)00070-7; Lisa Allen-Hall et al., "*Uncaria Ttmentosa* acts as a potent TNF-α inhibitor through NF-κB," *Journal of Ethnopharmacology* 127, no. 3 (February 2010): 685–93, https://doi.org/10.1016/j.jep.2009.12.004; S. Lamm, Y. Sheng, and R. W. Pero, "Persistent Response to Pneumococcal Vaccine in Individuals Supplemented With a Novel Water Soluble Extract of Uncaria

Tomentosa, C-Med-100," *Phytomedicine* 8, no. 4 (July 2001): 267–74, https://doi.org/10.1078/0944-7113-00046.

52. T. Hutchison et al., "The Botanical Glycoside Oleandrin Inhibits Human T-Cell Leukemia Virus Type-1 Infectivity and Env-Dependent Virological Synapse Formation," *Journal of Antivirals and Antiretrovirals* 11, no. 2 (2019): 184, https://www.longdom.org/open-access/the-botanical-glycoside-oleandrin-inhibits-human-tcell-leukemia-virus-type1-infectivity-and-envdependent-virological-synapse-forma-44367.html.

53. "How to Avoid Flu Naturally," ImmuneHealthScience.com. See also Albert Sanchez et al., "Role of Sugars in Human Neutrophilic Phagocytosis," *American Journal of Clinical Nutrition* 26, no. 11 (November 1973): 1180–84, https://doi.org/10.1093/ajcn/26.11.1180.

CHAPTER 8

1. Tony Perkins, "One Church's Story of What Not to Do," Family Research Council, March 24, 2020, https://www.frc.org/get.cfm?i=WA20C48&f=WU20C15.

2. Mark Palenske, "I know that some of you have wished for another update sooner than this, but sitting down at the computer is not my highest priority at this point....," Facebook, March 22, 2020, 6:25 p.m., https://www.facebook.com/mark.palenske/posts/2833351696745508.

3. Perkins, "One Church's Story of What Not to Do."

4. Tales Azzoni and Andrew Dampf, "Game Zero: Spread of Virus Linked to Champions League Match," Associated Press, March 25, 2020, https://apnews.com/ae59cfc0641fc63afd09182bb832ebe2; Samantha Hawley, "Coronavirus in Spain Is 'Frightening on Every Level.' So How Did Things Get So Bad There?," ABC, updated March 31, 2020, https://www.abc.net.au/news/2020-04-01/spains-coronavirus-reality-is-grim-how-did-it-start-there/12103590.

5. Erika Edwards, "Not Just Older People: Younger Adults Are Also Getting the Coronavirus," NBC Universal, March 17, 2020, https://www.nbcnews.com/health/health-news/not-just-older-people-younger-adults-are-also-getting-coronavirus-n1160416.

6. Píen Huang, "How Coronavirus Spreads: A Cough in Your Face....Or a Kiss on Your Cheek," NPR, March 5, 2020, https://www.npr.org/sections/goatsandsoda/2020/03/05/812570693/

how-coronavirus-spreads-a-cough-in-your-face-or-a-kiss-on-your-cheek.

7. Alexandra Topping and Nadeem Badshah, "Coronavirus: New UK and Mallorcan Cases Linked to French Ski Resort Cluster," *Guardian*, February 10, 2020, https://www.theguardian.com/world/2020/feb/09/fourth-person-in-uk-tests-positive-for-coronavirus.

8. Matthew Karnitschnig, "The Austrian Ski Town That Spread Coronavirus Across the Continent," Politico, updated March 20, 2020, https://www.politico.eu/article/the-austrian-ski-town-that-spread-coronavirus-across-the-continent/.

9. Miranda Bryant, "Coronavirus Spread at Rikers Is a 'Public Health Disaster,' Says Jail's Top Doctor," *Guardian*, April 1, 2020, https://www.theguardian.com/us-news/2020/apr/01/rikers-island-jail-coronavirus-public-health-disaster.

10. Steve Orr, "Wife Sick After Husband Hid Coronavirus Symptoms to Visit Her in the Maternity Ward," *USA Today*, updated March 31, 2020, https://www.usatoday.com/story/news/nation/2020/03/31/coronavirus-dad-hides-symptoms-gain-access-ny-maternity-ward/5093274002/.

11. S. I. McMillen and David E. Stern, *None of These Diseases: The Bible's Health Secrets for the 21st Century* (Grand Rapids, MI: Revell, 2008), 17–21, https://www.amazon.com/None-These-Diseases-Secrets-Century/dp/080075719X.

12. McMillen and Stern, *None of These Diseases*. See also *Encyclopaedia Britannica*, s.v. "Ignaz Semmelweis," updated March 26, 2020, https://www.britannica.com/biography/Ignaz-Semmelweis.

13. Lydia Bourouiba, "A Sneeze," *New England Journal of Medicine* 375 (2016): e15, https://doi.org/10.1056/NEJMicm1501197.

14. Fuhrman, *Super Immunity*, 54.

15. Richard Read, "Choir Practice Turns Fatal. Airborne Coronavirus Strongly Suspected," *Los Angeles Times*, March 29, 2020, https://www.latimes.com/world-nation/story/2020-03-29/coronavirus-choir-outbreak.

16. Dave Birkett, "Ex-Michigan Football's Mark Campbell Is Coronavirus Cautionary Tale," *Detroit Free Press*, April 7, 2020, https://www.freep.com/story/sports/nfl/lions/2020/04/07/michigan-football-mark-campbell-coronavirus-nfl/2956106001/.

17. Mayo Clinic Staff, "Hand-Washing: Do's and Don'ts," Mayo Clinic, accessed May 4, 2020, https://www.mayoclinic.org/healthy-lifestyle/adult-health/in-depth/hand-washing/art-20046253.

18. Sabrina Stierwalt, "Does Soap Really Kill 99.9% of Germs?," Quick and Dirty Tips, June 13, 2016, https://www.quickanddirtytips.com/education/science/does-soap-really-kill-999-of-germs.

19. Pall Thordarson, "The Science of Soap—Here's How It Kills the Coronavirus," *Guardian*, March 12, 2020, https://www.theguardian.com/commentisfree/2020/mar/12/science-soap-kills-coronavirus-alcohol-based-disinfectants.

20. Brenda Goodman, "The Power of Hand-Washing to Prevent Coronavirus," WebMD, March 6, 2020, https://www.webmd.com/lung/news/20200306/power-of-hand-washing-to-prevent-coronavirus.

21. Goodman, "The Power of Hand-Washing to Prevent Coronavirus."

22. Barry, *The Great Influenza*, 311.

CHAPTER 9

1. Amanda Roberts, "'Don't Take It Lightly,': Unlikely Coronavirus Survivor's Story and Message for Others," Fox 8, updated April 1, 2020, https://www.fox8live.com/2020/04/01/dont-take-it-lightly-unlikely-coronavirus-survivors-story-message-others/.

2. Roberts, "'Don't Take It Lightly.'"

3. Alexandria Hein, "Recovered Coronavirus Patient's Message to ICU Staff Goes Viral: 'You Are All Rockstars,'" FOX News, March 25, 2020, https://www.foxnews.com/health/recovered-coronavirus-patients-message-goes-viral.

4. Fuhrman, *Super Immunity*, 46.

CHAPTER 10

1. Mike Evans, "A Special Word From Dr. Mike Evans," Jerusalem Prayer Team, accessed May 4, 2020, http://pages.jerusalemprayerteam.org/2020-Coronavirus-Great-Awakening_2020-Coronavirus-Great-Awakening-LP-ALL.html?fbclid=IwAR2Sei68Jx14eI-I2BBTswgcU6N9dsZXGoagibsMRJJWJ9OKqk8U49UE9tA.

2. Streams Ministries, "The Coming Perfect Storm (Full)," YouTube, July 27, 2016, https://www.youtube.com/watch?v=kzPJjOzZorg&feature=emb_title.

3. Streams Ministries, "The Coming Perfect Storm (Full)."

4. Streams Ministries, "The Coming Perfect Storm (Full)."

5. Anne Graham Lotz, "Is There a Blessing in the Coronavirus?," Anne Graham Lotz/AnGeL Ministries, March 23, 2020, https://www.annegrahamlotz.org/2020/03/23/is-there-a-blessing-in-the-coronavirus/.

6. Lotz, "Is There a Blessing in the Coronavirus?"

7. Lotz, "Is There a Blessing in the Coronavirus?"

8. Lotz, "Is There a Blessing in the Coronavirus?"

9. Lotz, "Is There a Blessing in the Coronavirus?"

10. Chuck Pierce, "Chuck Pierce Prophesies: 'Massive Plague-Like Invasion' Will Test Us Through Passover," Charisma News, March 22, 2020, https://www.charismanews.com/opinion/80444-chuck-pierce-prophesies-massive-plague-like-invasion-will-test-us-through-passover.

11. Pierce, "Chuck Pierce Prophesies."

APPENDIX C

1. Information adapted from Walgreens.